Report of Investigations 9691

A NEW PERIMETER CONTROL BLAST DESIGN CONCEPT FOR UNDERGROUND METAL/NONMETAL DRIFTING APPLICATIONS

Stephen R. Iverson, William A. Hustrulid, and Jeffrey C. Johnson

DEPARTMENT OF HEALTH AND HUMAN SERVICES
Centers for Disease Control and Prevention
National Institute for Occupational Safety and Health
Office of Mine Safety and Health Research
Pittsburgh, PA • Spokane, WA

March 2013

Disclaimer

Mention of any company or product does not constitute endorsement by the National Institute for Occupational Safety and Health (NIOSH). In addition, citations to Web sites external to NIOSH do not constitute NIOSH endorsement of the sponsoring organizations or their programs or products. Furthermore, NIOSH is not responsible for the content of these Web sites. All Web addresses referenced in this document were accessible as of the publication date.

Ordering Information

To receive documents or other information about occupational safety and health topics, contact NIOSH at

Telephone: **1–800–CDC–INFO** (1–800–232–4636)
TTY: 1–888–232–6348
e-mail: cdcinfo@cdc.gov

or visit the NIOSH Web site at **www.cdc.gov/niosh**.

For a monthly update on news at NIOSH, subscribe to NIOSH *eNews* by visiting **www.cdc.gov/niosh/eNews**.

DHHS (NIOSH) Publication No. 2013–129

March 2013

Table of Contents

Figures

Tables

ACRONYMS AND ABBREVIATIONS

ANFO	Ammonium Nitrate Fuel Oil
CSL	Crosshole sonic logging
MAE	Modified Ash Energy
MSHA	Mine Safety and Health Administration
MVP	Micro-velocity probe
NIOSH	National Institute for Occupational Safety and Health
P-wave	Compressional wave
PETN	Pentaerythritol tetranitrate
PPV	Peak particle velocity
RBS	Relative bulk strength
RMR	Rock Mass Rating
RWS	Relative weight strength
S-wave	Shear wave
SSE	Solids stabilized emulsion
UCS	Uniaxial compressive strength
VOD	Velocity of detonation

UNIT OF MEASURE ABBREVIATIONS

%	percent
μsec	microsecond
atm	atmosphere
cm	centimeter
cm^3	cubic centimeter
cm^3/g	cubic centimeter per gram
°C	degree Celsius
g	gram
g/cm^3	gram per cubic centimeter
GPa	gigapascal
K	Kelvin
kcal/kg	kilocalories per kilogram
kg	kilogram
kg/m	kilogram per meter
kg/m^3	kilogram per cubic meter
km/sec	kilometer per second
L/kg	liter per kilogram
m	meter
MHz	megahertz
MJ/kg	megajoules per kilogram
mm	millimeter
MPa	megapascals
ms	millisecond
m/sec	meters per second
m^2	square meter
m^3	cubic meter
m^3/m	cubic meter per meter
sec	second

A NEW PERIMETER CONTROL BLAST DESIGN CONCEPT FOR UNDERGROUND METAL/NONMETAL DRIFTING APPLICATIONS

Stephen R. Iverson, William A. Hustrulid, and Jeffrey C. Johnson

Office of Mine Safety and Health Research
National Institute for Occupational Safety and Health

Abstract

This report presents a new concept in perimeter control blasting for underground metal/nonmetal mine drifting applications focusing on the importance of the buffer holes in a blast design. The new blast design concept applies the understanding of radial damage that is caused by the buffer hole column charge. Buffer hole radial damage is defined by a practical damage limit applied to the rock lying between the buffer holes and the perimeter. A favorable comparison was made between five successful controlled blast designs and the concept of practical damage limit. This concept is easy to use and acceptance of the approach would only require mines to conduct trial blasts to test the design theory.

Introduction

Drift driving is an important part of bringing metal/nonmetal mines into operation. Drifting provides access to an orebody for openings such as main haulage ways, main levels, ramps, crosscuts, sublevels, etc. The width, height, cross-sectional shape, and length of a drift depend on the use of the various mine openings. The typical method of drifting is to drill and blast. Blasting is an economical method to break rock, but the consequence of blasting is damage to the perimeter of the opening. The damage results in overbreak or rock that was not designed to be removed, loose rock to be scaled, and permanent damage to the remaining perimeter. Both the lack of a controlled blast design and of precision drilling are the main causes of perimeter damage. Perimeter damage was assessed in 2006 and 2007 by researchers from the National Institute for Occupational Safety and Health (NIOSH) during field investigations of blasting practices at mines in the United States [Iverson et al. 2007; Warneke et al. 2007; McHugh et al. 2008a; McHugh et al. 2008b]. It was found that mines were drilling blastholes without precision drills and at best were only able to maintain parallel blasthole orientations. Further, the blast designs were based primarily on miners' experience and capabilities. The results were a wide range of blast patterns, cut designs, hole spacings for the perimeters, the number of empty holes and spacing for line drilling, perimeter burdens, explosive types used, use of perimeter hole decoupling to prevent damage, blast round length, and variability in cross-sectional arch design and implementation.

The field investigations into drifting practices were important to outline safety problems linked to ground control. The obvious safety problems are:

- Overbreak results in wider spans that require additional ground support and an increased likelihood of failure if not properly assessed.

- Rough and undulating back and wall surfaces occur due to aggressive blasting and likely increase the hazards associated with scaling and the installation of bolts and support accessories.

- Lack of perimeter control by aggressive blasting will damage the perimeter to the point where more scaling is required and more potential loose rock could develop.

- Flat-arched backs impose additional bolting requirements where a rounded arch will typically aid in supporting the back.

Mine Safety and Health Administration (MSHA) accident statistics were reviewed by NIOSH engineers in 2006 and it was determined that fall-of-ground accidents in metal and nonmetal mines could be further prevented by improving the blasting methods. Interaction with the mining community to identify critical hazards was completed through field investigations.

Blasting has a tremendous influence on roof and rib stability [Iannacchione and Prosser 1997]. Precision drilling technology and controlled blast designs are available to accomplish better blasting perimeter control. The latest technology in drill jumbos are computer controlled and can drill precision holes using an engineered design. Mines are beginning to use these drills, and the future will hold the results as to the benefits of these technologies and methods. The blast designs currently used at the majority of mines in the United States are less developed and are based on dated design methods. Current controlled blast designs are based on closely spaced perimeter holes using the blasthole diameter to determine the perimeter spacing and burden and are not based on the explosive quantity or type for the perimeter holes and do not consider the effect of perimeter damage by the buffer holes [Holmberg 1982; Konya 2006].

This report proposes for the mining community an easy-to-use blast design method that includes improvements for determining the perimeter burden based on the effect of damage from buffer holes. This means that the distance or burden between the perimeter holes and the next line of blastholes defined as the buffer holes is determined by the damage caused by the buffer hole detonations. The new design method also includes the concept of locating the perimeter holes in an alternating arrangement in relation to the buffer hole locations.

The research and development of the new design described in this report was aimed at:

- Identifying the effectiveness of perimeter control in current drift designs
- Conducting experiments to determine the blast damage extent and factors influencing damage
- Studying blast damage models
- Packaging the blast damage models into an engineer and miner friendly design concept

This report includes:

- An introduction to the new perimeter control design philosophy and concept
- A blast damage model for calculating practical damage
- An evaluation of single hole blasts conducted in large concrete blocks to understand radial crack damage
- A description of five successful design examples demonstrating application of the design concept

Simple assumptions (that the rock mass is homogenous, isotropic, and a structure-free rock mass) are made in regards to drift design to focus on the importance of the practical damage limit and buffer row placement. Future research will be needed to address rock structure, detonation timing and sequencing, the interaction between adjacent holes detonated in a design, and the potential for improvements in fragmentation and perimeter control using electric detonators.

The Practical Damage Radius

Background

Perimeter control blasting is commonly applied to the roof but increasingly it is being applied to the walls as well. Figure 1 illustrates the different design sectors as distinguished by Holmberg [1982] for a drift round.

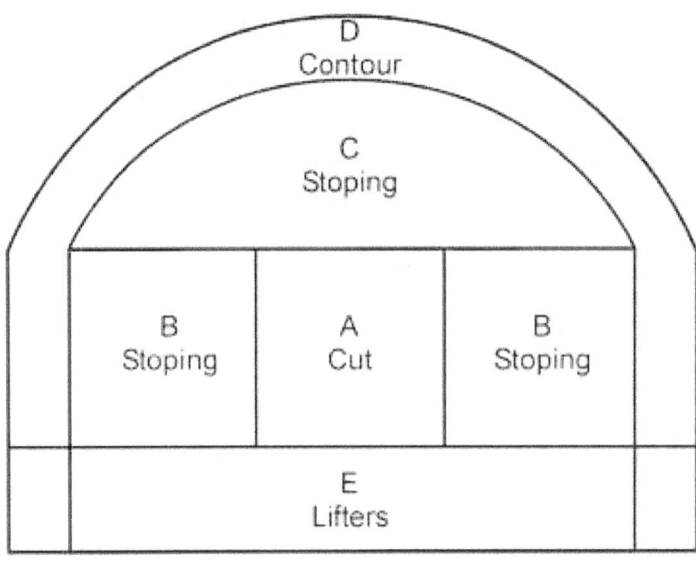

Figure 1. Diagrammatic representation of the design sectors involved in a drift round. After Holmberg [1982].

To better understand the traditional approach to perimeter control, the following is a description of the Holmberg [1982] algorithm. One begins by designing the cut, the contour, and the lifter sectors. When the particular designs for each of the sectors have been completed, they are added to the overall drift design. The so-called stoping holes are then added as needed. The implication is that the holes/explosives included in the different sectors are responsible for removing the associated rock. In the example shown in Figure 2 the width ("burden") of the contour sector is denoted as B. Particularly in hard, strong rock it is expected that the amount of explosive charge required to remove the contour sector of rock is quite high, and this subsequently would place quite strong requirements on the perimeter row design. For the Holmberg design, the contour (perimeter) burden is simply determined based on the spacing of the perimeter holes using:

$$B = 1.25E \tag{1}$$

where B = perimeter burden (m),
E = perimeter hole spacing (m),

and

$$E = kd \tag{2}$$

where k = 15 to 16, and
d = perimeter blasthole diameter (m).

Holmberg [1982] suggests analysis of the stoping, buffer, and perimeter holes for perimeter damage using critical peak particle velocity (PPV). The damage extent is illustrated in Figure 3.

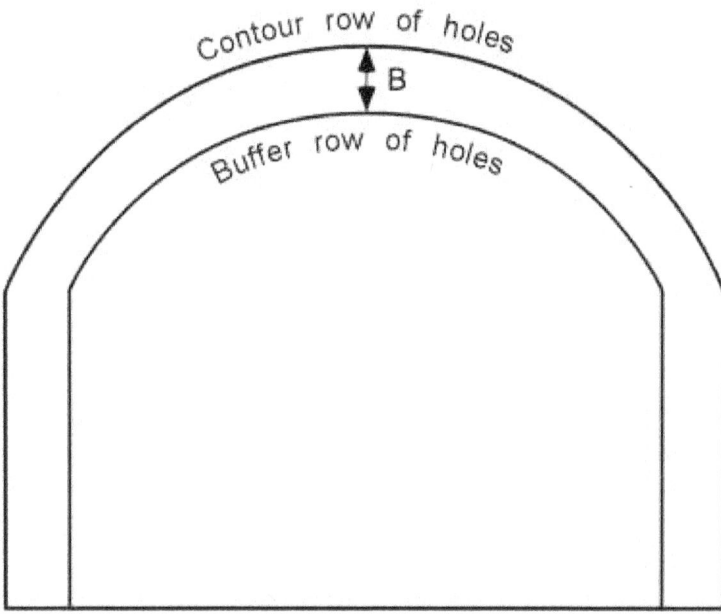

Figure 2. Contour sector bounded by the contour row and the buffer row.

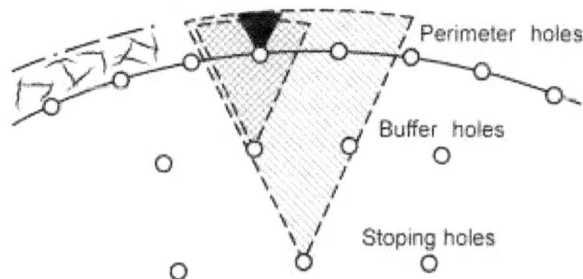

Figure 3. The charge concentrations in the holes close to the contour are adjusted so that the damage zone from each hole coincides with the expected crack limit. After Holmberg [1982].

Figure 3 shows potential contributions of the perimeter, buffer holes, and stoping holes in breaking the contour sector of rock and eventually damaging the perimeter rock. Not surprisingly, these contributions precondition the rock towards the perimeter. This is supported by Tesarik et al. [2011] who found through analysis of peak particle velocities that blast damage occurs beyond the subsequent row to be detonated. Preconditioning is a common phenomenon where blasting fragmentation results in weakening the fragments by microcracking [McCarter, 1996].

Buffer Holes in Practical Design

Buffer holes have previously been suggested for use in blast design as described by Hustrulid and Johnson [2008]. A practical damage radius (R_d) is determined for each blasthole/explosive combination. The damage radius calculated from the buffer holes would determine the perimeter burden. By "practical," it is meant that if the rock mass lying outside of this ring were removed, the rock remaining within the ring would easily break apart. As can be seen in Figure 4, the practical damage zone consists of both crushing and cracking components. The idea is to design the buffer holes so that their associated damage radius extends to the desired drift perimeter where the practical damage radius:

$$R_d = B \tag{3}$$

where R_d = practical damage radius, and
 B = contour row burden.

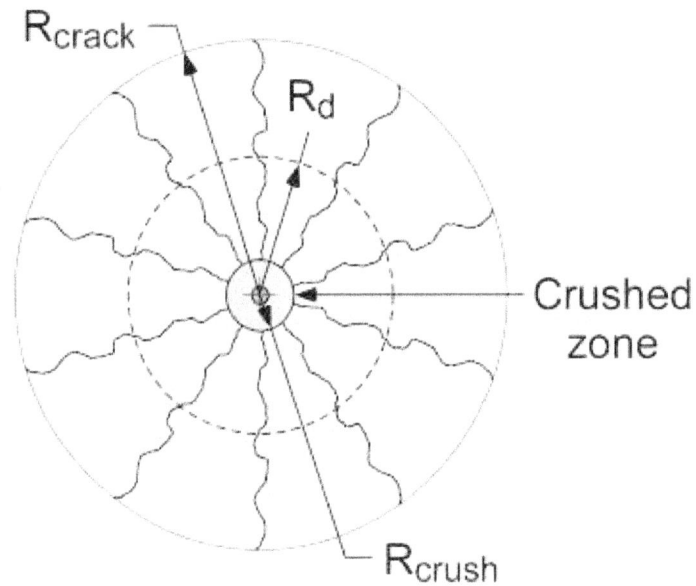

**Figure 4. Diagrammatic representation of the crushed, cracked, and
damaged zones surrounding a blasthole.**

It is logical to consider the extent of the damage surrounding a cylindrical charge to be a function of the available explosive energy, or the pressure applied to the wall of the blasthole. In reality, it is most probably a combination of both. In reviewing Figure 4, three different limits can be considered:

- crushing
- cracking
- practical damage

6

Holmberg and Persson [1979] offered a practical approach in determining the cracking limit through their well-known design curves relating the PPV, radius, and the explosive charge concentration. Referring back to Figure 3, the graphic visually presents Holmberg and Persson's damage concept that the crack radii from the buffer and stoping rows of holes should not exceed that associated with the contour holes. When circles are drawn in the figure rather than simply arcs, one can easily visualize that the representation is consistent with the proposed practical damage radius approach to design (Figure 5). It must be emphasized, however, that the PPV approach is based on the cracking radius rather than on the practical damage radius. Figure 6 provides a visual representation of the smaller practical damage limit applied to the buffer holes for the same diagram.

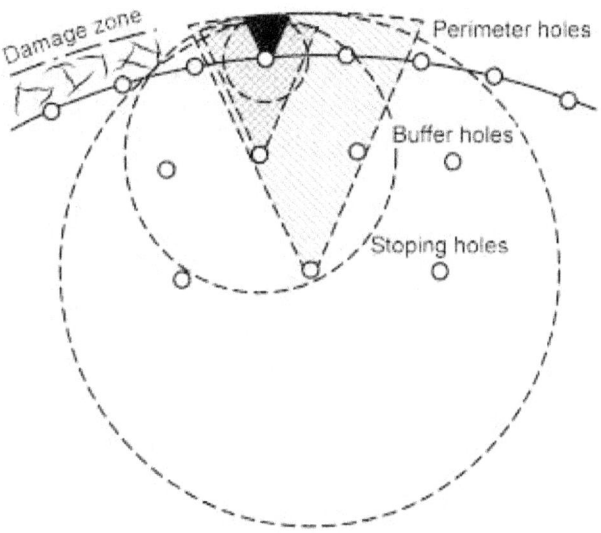

Figure 5. Radial crack damage circles applied to holes emphasized in the Holmberg [1982] perimeter damage extent diagram.

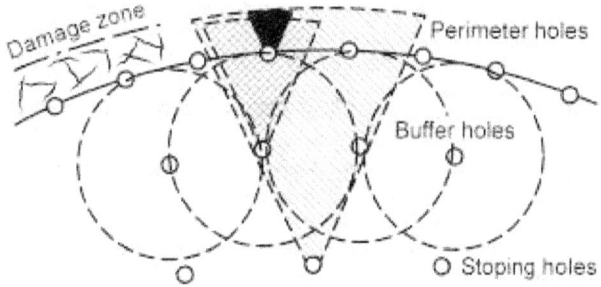

Figure 6. Practical damage circles only applied to buffer holes in the Holmberg [1982] perimeter damage extent diagram.

In some cases, for example in tunnel construction, the cracking radius is of prime concern and must be carefully controlled. In most cases, however, the primary control is on the size and shape of the excavation as denoted by the excavation limits. In design, one then utilizes, first and foremost, the practical damage limit. One can estimate the expected cracking limits but this is done more for interest than as a control. Through the use of presplitting of the perimeter row one can, at least in principle, control both the cracking limits and the excavation limits.

Modified Ash Energy (MAE) Approach

Background

In 1963, Ash [1963a,b,c,d] published his now-classic papers dealing with blast design in open pit mines and quarries. Figure 7 below is an isometric representation of two blastholes from a typical open pit mine or quarry and shows Ash's various design parameters.

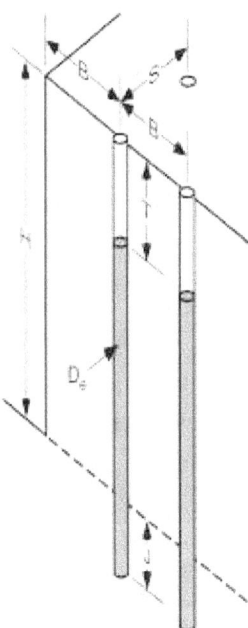

Figure 7. Isometric view of Ash's blast design parameters [Ash 1963a,b,c,d].

Using field data collected from a large number of operations, Ash [1963a,b,c,d] summarized the different design parameters. If these design parameters are applied to underground blast design, these same parameters should apply. He found that the subdrill (J), the stemming (T), the spacing (S) and the bench height, and the expected excavation length (H) could all be related to the burden (B). Most importantly, he found that for fully charged holes the burden (B) was related to the blasthole diameter (D_e) as shown in the following equation:

$$B = K_B D_e \tag{4}$$

where B = burden,
K_B = constant, and
D_e = hole diameter.

The value of K_B can vary with both the rock and the explosive, though Ash recommends that for average rock conditions $K_B = 30$ except when using a lighter density charge of field-mixed aluminum nitrate fuel oil (ANFO) where K_B is reduced to a range of 20 to 25. Hustrulid [1999a] found that $K_B = 25$ when using ANFO at a density of 0.80 g/cm^3 in rock of medium density (2.65 g/cm^3).

Ash's work has very successfully captured the experience in blasting. The ratios are largely followed today with the possible exception of the hole spacing relationship. Further, the range of rock types, explosive types, and blasthole diameters examined by Ash provide a satisfactory empirical analysis for conditions and ranges also found in underground mines. Ash contends that K_B can be modified using explosive density and rock density to values as small as 20 and as high as 40. This range of K_B would be the limitation of its use for determining burden. Ash suggests a practical range for both explosive densities and rock densities. [Ash 1963a,b,c,d].

Equation

Hustrulid [1999a] proposed a design procedure based on energy coverage. It was assumed that the holes were charged fully coupled. The radius of the damage circle used in this approach was obtained by equating available explosive energy to that required to produce acceptable fragmentation. In this regard, it was assumed that the use of ANFO with density 0.85 g/cm^3 to blast an average rock of density 2.65 g/cm^3 yielded satisfactory results when $K_B = 25$. The formula expressing the ratio K_B for other rock-explosive combinations becomes:

$$K_B = 25 \sqrt{\frac{\rho_e \, s_{ANFO}}{\rho_{ANFO} s_{1ANFO}}} \sqrt{\frac{2.65}{\rho_r}} \tag{5}$$

where ρ_e = density of the explosive used (g/cm^3),
s_{ANFO} = weight strength of the explosive relative to ANFO,
ρ_{ANFO} = density of ANFO = 0.85 g/cm^3,
s_{1ANFO} = weight strength of ANFO relative to ANFO = 1, and
ρ_r = density of the rock mass (g/cm^3).

This formula described originally in Hustrulid and Johnson [2008] provides a value of K_B which follows the Ash [1963a,b,c,d] and Hustrulid [1999a] recommendations regarding the effect of explosive energy and rock density. Based simply on the geometry of just-touching damage circles,

$$B = 2R_d \tag{6}$$

The basic Ash [1963a,b,c,d] burden formula becomes

$$B = 2R_d = K_B D_e = K_B 2r_h \qquad (7)$$

where r_h = hole radius, and
           R_d = damage radius.

From Equations 6 and 7, it follows that

$$2R_d = K_B 2r_h \ \ or \ \ R_d = K_B r_h \qquad (8)$$

Finally, one obtains the relationship

$$\frac{R_d}{r_h} = 25\sqrt{\frac{\rho_e \, S_{ANFO}}{\rho_{ANFO}}} \sqrt{\frac{2.65}{\rho_r}} \qquad (9)$$

It is recognized that

$$\frac{\rho_e \, S_{ANFO}}{\rho_{ANFO}} = RBS \qquad (10)$$

where RBS = bulk strength relative to ANFO.

The relative bulk strength (RBS) is often provided by explosive suppliers. Thus Equation 10 becomes

$$\frac{R_d}{r_h} = 25\sqrt{RBS} \sqrt{\frac{2.65}{\rho_r}} \qquad (11)$$

As can be seen, the approach is quite simple involving available explosive properties and the density of the rock as inputs. Thus, this approach is attractive for mine application.

Calculation Examples

An explosive properties dataset of 15 types was evaluated as applied to a 48-mm-diameter blasthole. The dataset is shown in Table 1 and plotted in Figure 8. Ash suggests his K_B value can be modified based on a range of rock densities from 2.2 g/cm^3 to 3.2 g/cm^3. A rock density of 2.7 g/cm^3 was considered most common. Lighter charges will have a lower K_B while heavier charges will have a larger K_B. This is equally true with the R_d/r_h ratio in Figure 8 where the lighter charges are in the range of 25 and the heavier charges are closer to 30. A range of rock densities from 2.2 g/cm^3 to 3.2 g/cm^3 as described by Ash was applied, and the rock densities are shown as separate curves in Figure 8. [Ash 1963a,b,c,d].

Table 1. Selected explosives, properties, and calculated R_d/r_h damage results for a range of rock densities

Explosive	RBS	2.2	2.5	2.7	2.9	3.2
Orica Titan SSE*	0.66	22.3	21.0	20.2	19.5	18.5
Orica Titan SSE	0.70	23.0	21.6	20.8	20.0	19.1
Orica Titan SSE	0.74	23.6	22.2	21.3	20.6	19.6
Orica Titan SSE	0.78	24.2	22.7	21.9	21.1	20.1
Orica Titan SSE	0.82	24.8	23.3	22.4	21.6	20.6
Orica Titan SSE	0.86	25.4	23.8	22.9	22.1	21.1
Orica Titan SSE	0.90	26.0	24.4	23.5	22.6	21.5
DYNO MIX	0.92	26.3	24.6	23.7	22.9	21.8
Orica Titan SSE	0.94	26.5	24.9	24.0	23.1	22.0
DYNO Titan 7000	0.94	26.5	24.9	24.0	23.1	22.0
DYNO BlastEX	1.06	28.2	26.5	25.5	24.6	23.4
Orica Amex	1.10	28.8	27.0	26.0	25.1	23.9
DYNO BlastEX Plus	1.15	29.4	27.6	26.5	25.6	24.4
DYNO AP (tamped)	1.24	30.6	28.7	27.6	26.6	25.3
Orica Senatel Magnafrac (tamped)	1.20	30.1	28.2	27.1	26.2	24.9

* Solids stabilized emulsion

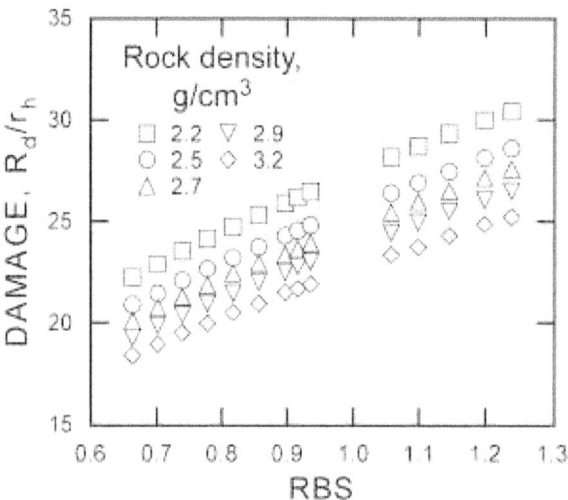

Figure 8. MAE practical damage R_d/r_h plot of selected explosives for a range of rock densities.

Other Damage Models Considered

Other damage methods for assigning a damage radius were investigated. These methods ranged from those that are empirically based to some with very solid theoretical roots. In theory or through support of other empirical datasets, some of the other damage models mentioned could be viable choices for determining the practical damage limit. The authors of this paper contend that the Modified Ash Energy (MAE) approach has the most comprehensive and empirically supported dataset and is based on commonly used explosives and rock properties. If one were to choose an approach for a first approximation of practical damage, it would be the MAE approach.

Short discussions on other damage models investigated for use in determining the practical damage radius are listed below:

- The Holmberg-Persson approach [Holmberg and Persson 1979] has been widely accepted and applied. In addition, by serving as a model for the development of other approaches, it has greatly contributed to advancing the field.

- The rock constant approach is based on work by Persson et al. [1994] where the rock constant c is the amount of explosive (kg/m^3) needed for breaking loose the rock at the toe in a defined blasting geometry. The rock constant ranges from 0.2 to 0.6. The rock constant equation for burden calculation can be found in Holmberg [1982] and in Persson et al. [1994].

- The modified Ash pressure model, as described in Hustrulid and Johnson [2008] and similar to the MAE model, was modified from work by Ash [1963a,b,c,d] and Hustrulid [1999a]. The RBS in the MAE approach is replaced with the explosion pressure. The explosion pressure is derived from an equation using explosive density and velocity of detonation (VOD).

- The Sher pressure-based approach to calculating blast damage is dependent on the explosive properties for calculating the explosion pressure and the calculation of damage based on the strength and elasticity of the rock mass [Sher 1997; Sher and Aleksandrova 1997; Sher and Aleksandrova 2007].

- The Drukovanyi approach is based on Drukovanyi et al. [1976] who presented a calculation for zones of fine crushing and radial fissures for exploding cylindrical charges.

- The Johnson model is based on the Hustrulid Bar test as described by Johnson [2010]. In this model, it was assumed that the damage radius was directly related to the damage done by the shock wave moving through the rock mass. The gas pressure was not considered.

- The Etkin approach is based on Etkin et al. [2001] that describes a calculation method for explosives selection and placement to protect the perimeter from damage. The Etkin approach is empirical in that a large amount of field data was collected to derive a blasting resistance factor and determination based on rock classification, joint spacing, and joint width. The Etkin approach is promising because it takes into account the rock structure.

- The Favreau approach is based on work by Favreau [1969] who presented a mathematical solution for the prediction of strain waves generated when a fully coupled explosive detonates inside a spherical cavity in an infinite, isotropic, homogeneous medium. These passing strain waves produce particle vibrations. The difficulty is in converting the spherical equation to a column charge equation. This was attempted using a string of elemental spheres that represent a column charge similar to the Holmberg-Persson approach.

- The Neiman approach pertains to a cylindrical charge as originally presented by Neiman [1979] but modified to take into account actual rock behavior and various explosives. The hydrodynamic approach was developed to predict the extent of blast damage caused by an explosive charge in an idealized rock mass as characterized by the peak particle velocity (PPV). A calibration factor was introduced to account for the actual behavior of the explosive in a particular rock mass. This factor is obtained by conducting a field test in which particle velocity measurements are made as a function of distance away from the charge [Tesarik and Hustrulid 2009].

13

Blast Damage Experiments

Blasting experiments were conducted in large concrete blocks that simulate rock [Iverson et al. 2009; Johnson 2010]. Results from these experiments were compared to the MAE practical damage limit R_d.

Experimental Methodology

The experimental method for assessing the damage level of the MAE R_d calculation is to have blocks with a range of rock densities and explosive RBS values to properly assess the range of rock densities and RBS values shown in Figure 8. The experiments that were conducted were limited to two types of emulsion and a narrow range of simulated rock densities. The damage results from the experiments could indicate a definite change in damage at the MAE R_d limit or at least provide better understanding of and quantify the damage at the R_d limit.

The experiments were explosive detonations in large concrete blocks and a blasthole of full-scale diameter, length, and radial extent. Full-scale tests best represent actual mine drifting conditions. The tests were comparable to actual drifting dimensions, explosives, and rock densities. A comparison of actual to experimental parameters is shown in Table 2.

Table 2. Comparison of experimental setup parameters to actual mine drifting parameters

Parameters	Mine drifting[*]	Block experiment
Diameter (mm)	44–48	38
Length (m)	2.4–3.7	1.2–1.8
Radial extent (m)	na†	2.6–3.6
Rock density (kg/m^3)	2,200–3,200	2,100–2,310
RBS	0.6–1.2	1.20–1.24

* Typical ranges of dimensions were found in field investigations and MAE input properties from Ash [1963a,b,c,d].

†na = not applicable

The explosive for the experiments was packaged emulsion. Emulsion provides uniformity in the explosive as compared to ANFO where the amount of pressure when pneumatically loading can result in varied in-place properties. The use of ANFO would also have required a larger hole diameter. The packaged emulsion was tamped to full coupling with the blasthole wall.

Damage was measured using various techniques including: (1) wire sawing to expose and measure the crack count and length, (2) seismic probes using inspection holes to determine the combined effect of microcrack damage and radial crack damage, and (3) measured strain applying the peak particle velocity (PPV) to relate the Holmberg-Persson [1979] damage limits to distance.

The analysis of the blocks included comparing the measured damage limits for each test to the MAE R_d for the specific simulated rock density and explosive properties. Finally, damage at the calculated MAE R_d practical damage limit was assessed.

The experimental design setups for blocks 1, 2, and 3 are shown in Figure 9, Figure 10, and Figure 11, respectively. The blastholes were 38 mm in diameter and drilled parallel to the free surface of each block. Three different burden dimensions and two brands of emulsion explosives were employed. The charges were fully coupled. The waves generated by the detonation process were measured at several distances away from the charge axis. The radial strain measurements collected from the embedded gages during the blast tests were converted to PPV. These were used to calculate PPV-distance curves to be related to the damage. The resulting radial cracks were observed on wire-sawn surface cuts made perpendicular to the charge column orientation. Postblast inspection holes were drilled into the damaged blocks. In-hole S-wave and crosshole P-wave velocities were measured. These measurements were used to determine if damage varied with distance from the charge. Preblast core samples were tested for static physical properties.

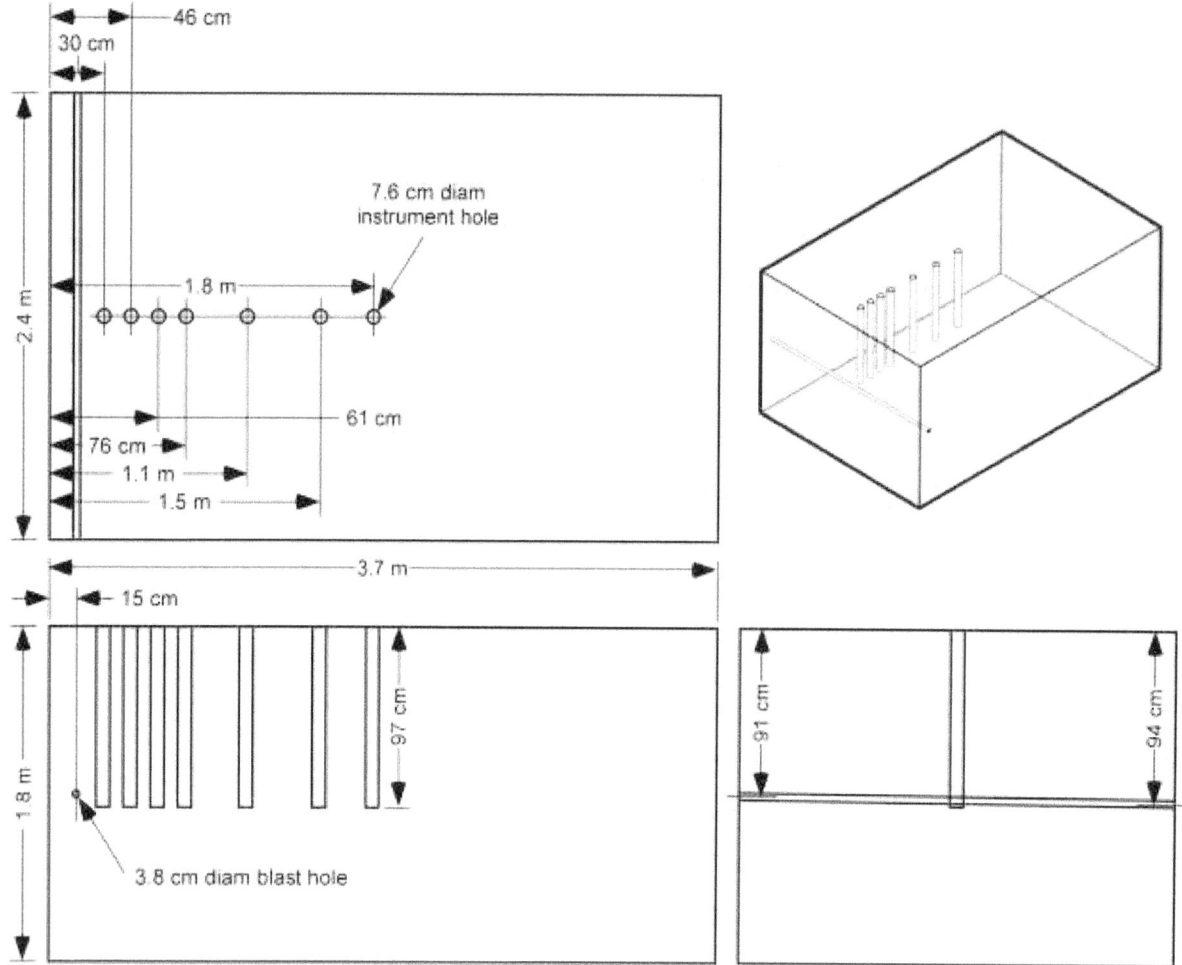

Figure 9. Engineering drawing of block 1 blasthole and strain gage sensor locations.

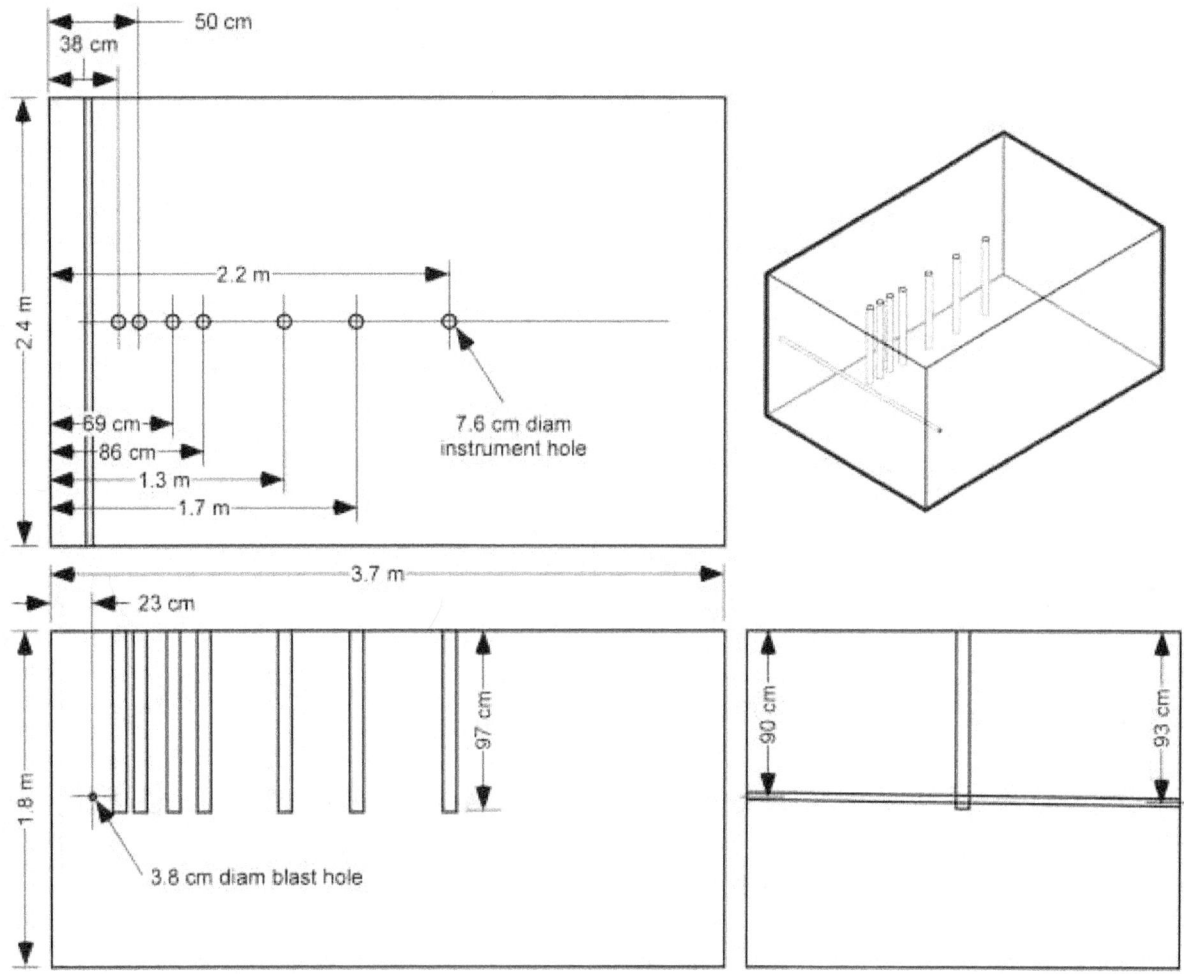

Figure 10. Engineering drawing of block 2 blasthole and strain gage sensor locations.

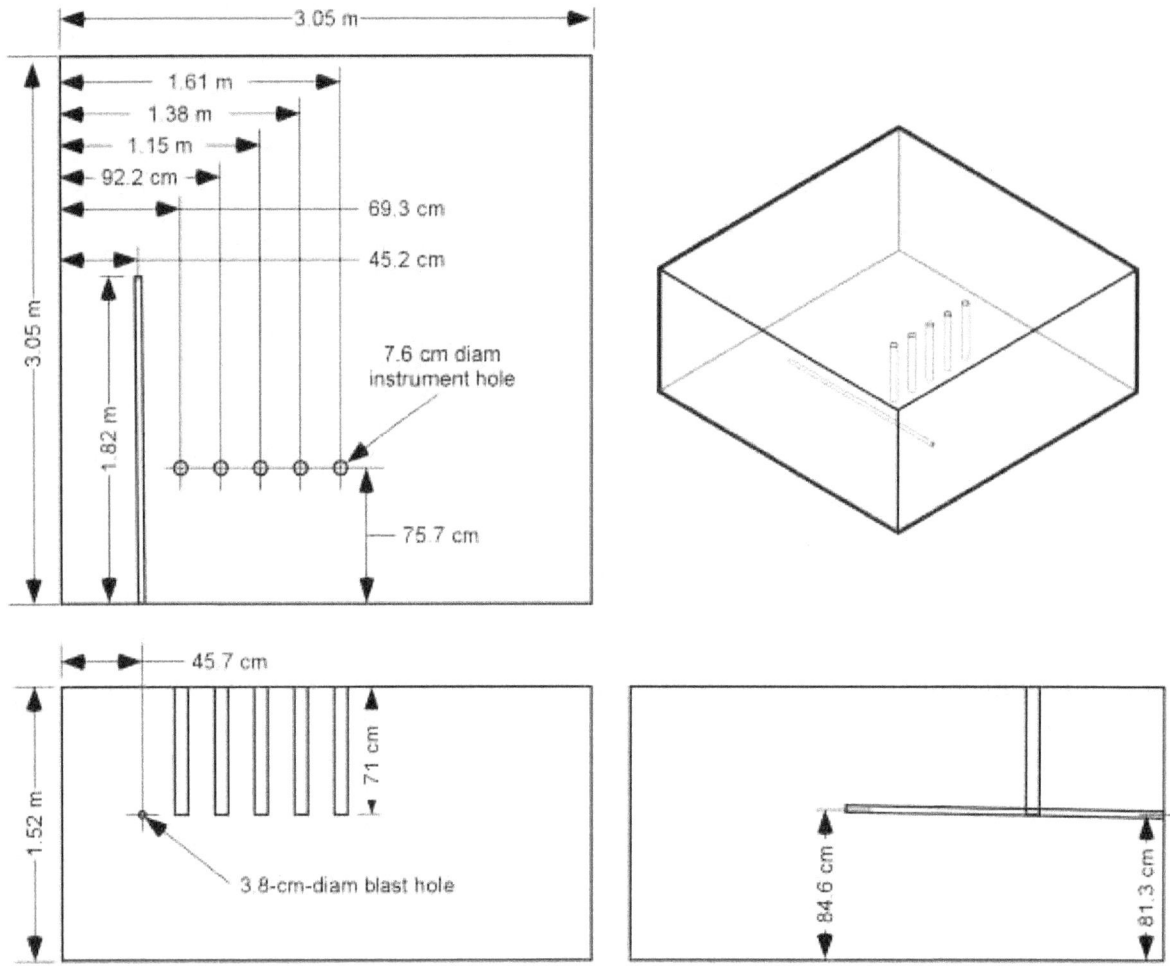

Figure 11. Engineering drawing of block 3 blasthole and strain gage sensor locations.

Test blocks 1 and 2 were 3.7 m long, 2.4 m wide, and 1.8 m high. Test block 3 was 3.0 m long by 3.0 m wide by 1.5 m high. All of the blastholes were drilled horizontally at mid-height and parallel to the short side of the block. Block 1 had a burden of 15 cm, block 2 had a burden of 23 cm, and block 3 had a burden of 46 cm.

In test blocks 1 and 2 the blastholes exited through the back of the block. Both ends of the blastholes were stemmed with 30 cm of clay. The resulting charged length was 1.8 m. In test block 3 the blasthole was drilled to a depth of 1.8 m and charged over a length of 1.2 m. The charge was not stemmed. Test block 1 as shown in the photograph in Figure 12 is prior to the blast experiment and shows the drilled blasthole and some of the fly rock barrier walls. Test block 2 as shown in the photograph in Figure 13 is after the blast experiment but before wire sawing to further expose the radial fracturing. Test block 3 as shown in a photograph in Figure 14 is during wire sawing to expose the radial fractures. Note that the grout columns are exposed from the access holes where the strain gages were located.

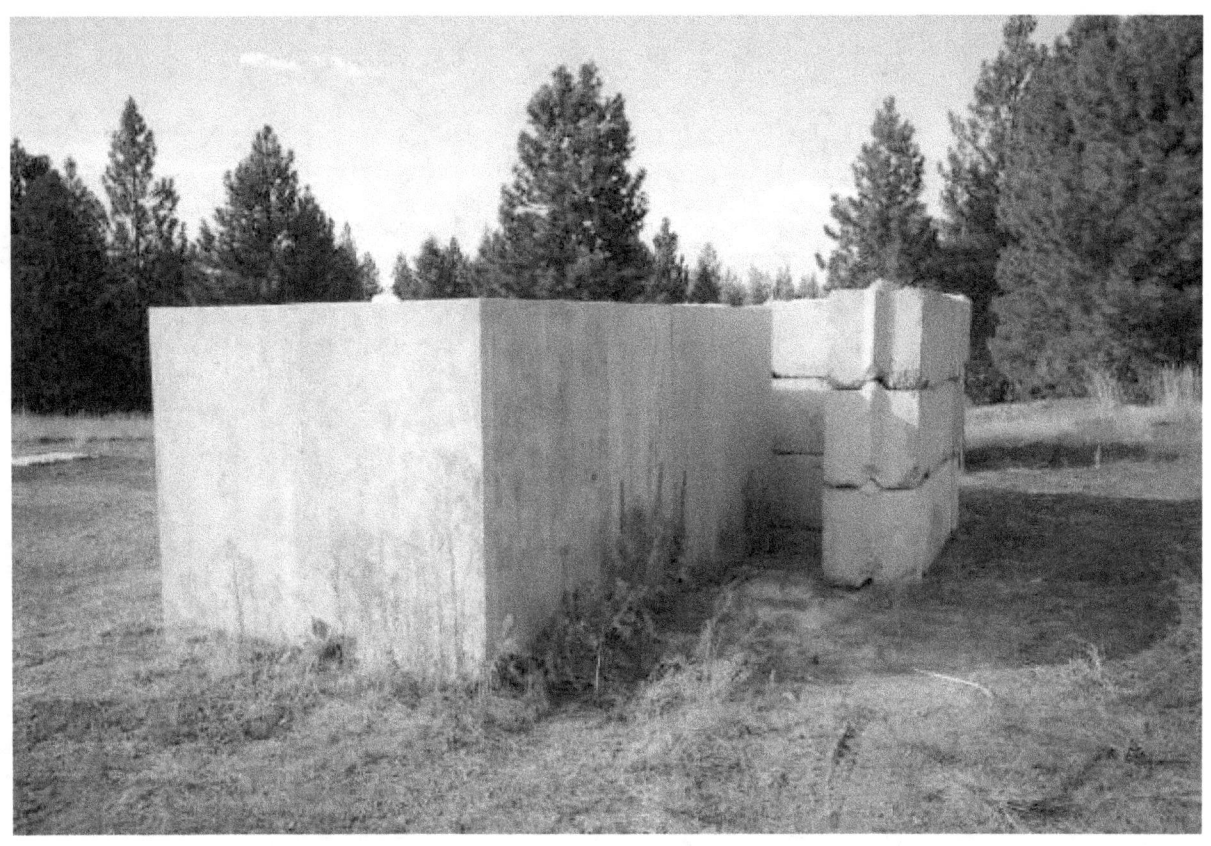

Figure 12. Block 1 prior to blasting showing flyrock barrier wall installed.

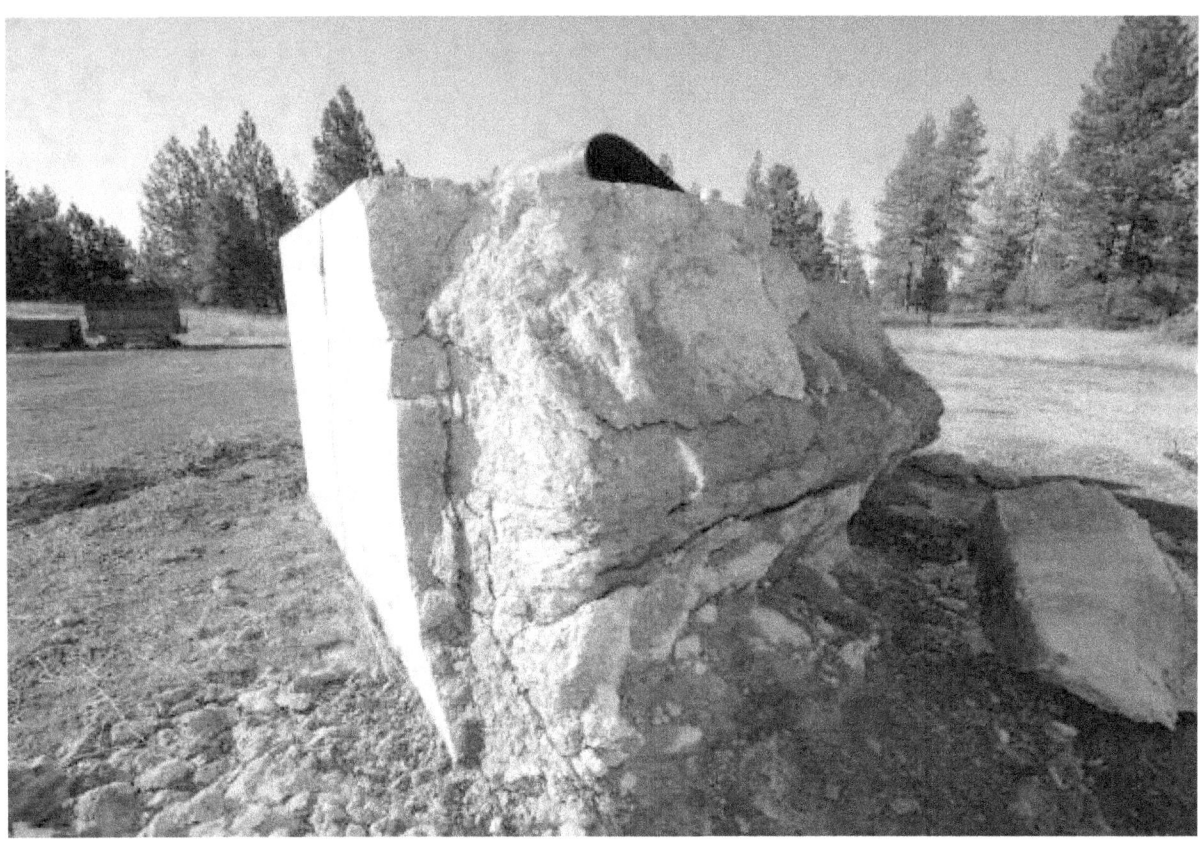

Figure 13. Block 2 after blasting and prior to wire sawing showing remnants of blasthole location.

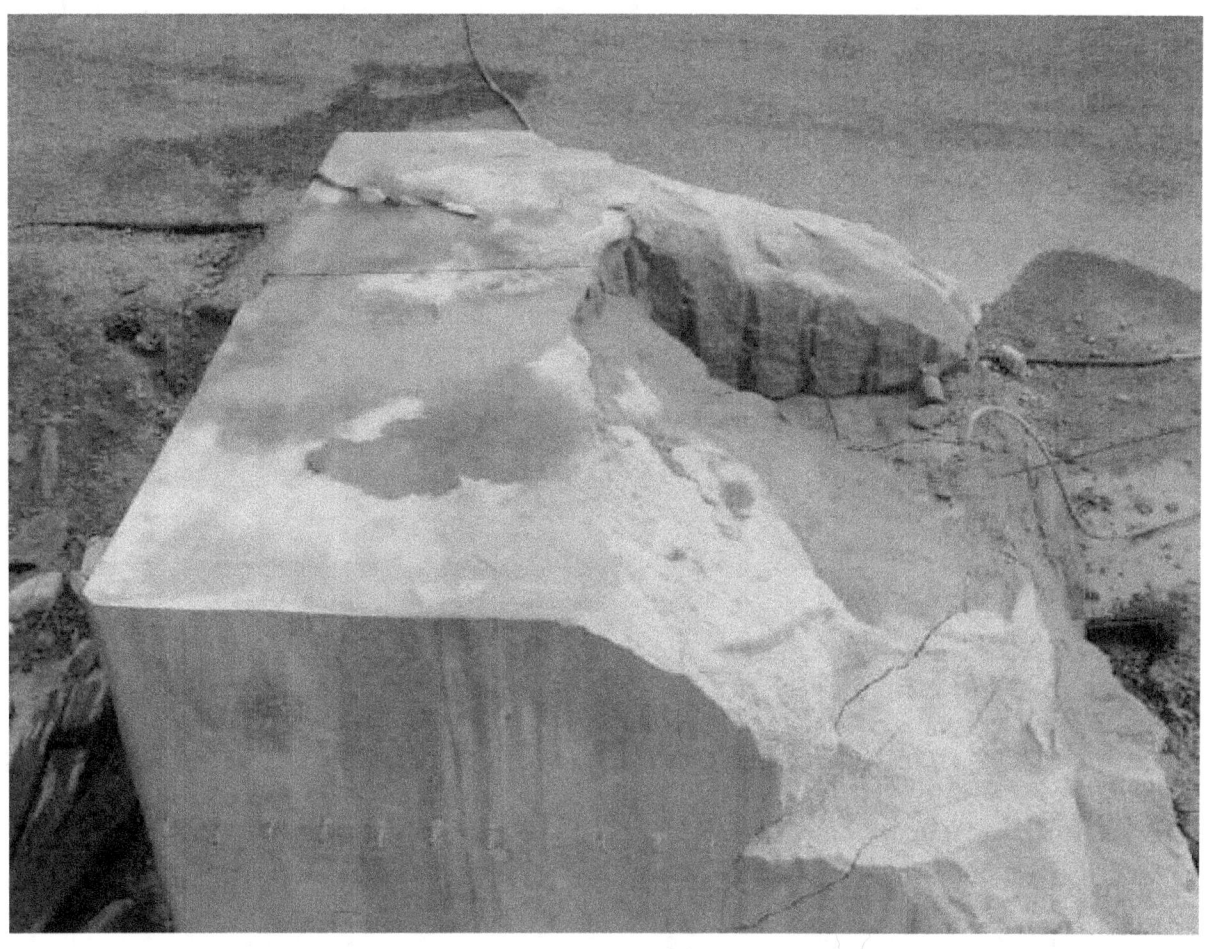

Figure 14. Block 3 during wire sawing to expose radial fractures.

Concrete Block and Explosive Properties

The concrete block properties as determined from cores extracted from the blocks are listed in Table 3.

Table 3. Concrete block properties tested

Property	Test block 1	Test block 2	Test block 3
Density (kg/m^3)	2,270	2,310	2,100
Unconfined compressive strength (MPa)	42	44	21
Brazilian tensile strength (MPa)	2.8	3.1	na*
Young's modulus (MPa)	29,500	32,000	13,100
Speed of sound (m/sec)	3,800	3,930	2,640

*na = not applicable

The Orica brand Senatel Magnafrac explosive was used in test blocks 1 and 2. The Dyno Nobel brand Dyno AP was the explosive used in test block 3 (block 3 was tested first and then followed by block 1 and block 2). The reason for changing to Senatel Magnafrac was that the Dyno AP explosive was no longer sold in small quantities. These stick explosives were considered fully coupled because tamping was performed after each stick was inserted (the first stick containing the detonator was not tamped). The published properties for these explosives are listed in Table 4.

Table 4. Explosive properties of the emulsions used in the blast experiments

Explosive Property	Dyno AP	Senatel Magnafrac
Density (kg/m^3)	1,150	1,110
Relative weight strength (RWS)	0.88	0.91
Relative bulk strength (RBS)	1.24	1.20

Micro-Velocity Probe

After blasting, 76-mm-diameter boreholes were collared and drilled into the blocks at one or more locations along the remaining half-barrel of the blastholes. The walls of these inspection holes were smooth and provided a good surface for making measurements using the Micro-Velocity Probe (MVP). This probe, in the form of a shuttle, is an S-wave generator and receiver. In this case, transmit-and-receive shoes were spaced at 10 cm. The first measurement was made with the MVP positioned just inside the collar and measurements were made at intervals of 2.5 cm. By observing the variation of S-wave velocity with depth, one obtains an indication of the extent of damage.

Crosshole Velocity Probes

The Crosshole Sonic Logging (CSL) testing method was used to evaluate the condition of the damaged block between pairs of parallel inspection holes. The inspection holes were collared on the remaining half-barrels and drilled horizontally and perpendicular. The CSL test involves filling the holes with water, inserting a pair of hydrophones into the parallel holes, and then simultaneously withdrawing the hydrophones by cables attached to a distance-measuring wheel while ultrasonic P-wave pulses are sent from the source hydrophone to the receiver hydrophone. The collars of the horizontal inspection holes were extended using plastic sleeves to provide a dam for maintaining water in the holes while testing. The system was set to send pulses every 1.3 cm as the hydrophones were pulled out. The test can be conducted quickly and the results easily analyzed. The CSL results are displayed as a plot of P-wave velocity versus distance into the boreholes. A decrease in the P-wave velocity of the block material between the boreholes near the blasthole is an indication of damage.

Wave Attenuation Measurements

A line of instrumentation holes oriented perpendicular to the charge axis was drilled from the top surface of each block for the purpose of monitoring the strain waves generated by the blast. The hole depth extended to the blasthole elevation. A specially prepared synthetic rock transducer to which four strain gages had been mounted (3 horizontal and 1 vertical) was then grouted at the bottom of each hole. The grout was of similar density and elasticity compared to the blocks, and strain waves were expected to pass through the grouted sensor locations. Of the three horizontal gages, one was mounted parallel to the charge axis, one perpendicular, and one at an angle of 45°. Data were collected at 1 MHz. Peak strain data from the horizontal gages that oriented perpendicular to the charge axis were plotted (Figure 15). The other strain orientations were not used in the presented damage models, thus they are not reported. From the regression curve fit, the radial strain values at a given distance are converted to peak particle velocity (PPV). The PPV values as presented by Persson et al. [1994] as they relate to damage were compared to the results. The damage limits and associated PPV values from Persson et al. are shown in Table 5 and include the Brazilian tensile strength limit from Johnson [2010]. Johnson found that the tensile strength of the Swedish Vanga granite was 20 MPa as tested using the splitting tensile strength method or twice the direct pull test value from Persson et al. [1994].

Table 5. PPV limits for blast damage types for hard gneiss or granite [Persson et al. 1994]

Damage type	Stress (MPa)	PPV (m/sec)	PPV factor relative to crushing
Crushing and compressive strength limit (150 MPa)	150	15	1
Good fragmentation	50	5	0.33
Fragmentation limit	25	2.5	0.17
Brazilian tensile strength limit (20 MPa)*	20	2.0	0.13
Incipient damage and direct pull tensile strength limit (10 MPa)	10	1.0	0.07
Incipient swelling	7	0.7	0.05

*Johnson [2010]

In Persson et al. [1994] the range of PPV damage values corresponds to a range of stress levels from 7 to 150 MPa. However, a factor is needed to compare the PPV damage limits to the much weaker experimental blocks. The PPV factors shown in Table 5 are proportional to the crushing PPV limit of 15 m/sec.

Now for comparison, the PPV damage limits are determined for the synthetic rocks of experimental blocks 1, 2, and 3. Table 6 shows the calculated crushing PPV damage limits and the factored estimates for the other damage limits for each block. The crushing PPV damage limits were calculated using the one-dimensional relationship for PPV and each block's compressive strength, speed of sound, and Young's modulus.

Table 6. Estimated Persson PPV damage limits for the experimental blocks using the compressive strength PPV factors [Persson et al. 1994]

Damage type	Block 1 PPV (m/sec)	Block 2 PPV (m/sec)	Block 3 PPV (m/sec)
Crushing	5.4	5.2	4.5
Good fragmentation	1.8	1.7	1.5
Fragmentation limit	0.92	0.90	0.77
Brazilian tensile strength limit	0.70	0.68	0.58
Incipient damage	0.38	0.36	0.32
Incipient swelling	0.27	0.26	0.23

The strain measurements will be plotted as strain vs. distance, and radial measurements of the estimated Persson PPV damage limits will be determined from the plot.

Additionally, material specimens were extracted from the experimental blocks to determine the dynamic compressive strength based on work by Johnson [2010] using the Hustrulid Bar experiment. The seismic limit testing on block 3 is described in Johnson [2010], and a similar test was later conducted on block 1. The bar test results from block 1 were a seismic limit strain of 0.002 and a dynamic compressive strength of 59 MPa. The expected PPV damage limit was determined to be 7.6 m/sec based on a speed of sound velocity of 3,800 m/sec. The bar test results from block 3 indicated a seismic limit strain of 0.0016 and a dynamic compressive strength of 21 MPa [Johnson 2010]. The expected PPV damage limit was determined to be at a PPV of 4.5 m/sec. The PPV was determined using a sound velocity of 2,800 m/sec. The seismic limit distance is determined from a plot of measured strain converted to PPV vs. distance and compared to the MAE practical damage limit.

Visual Assessment of Radial Crack Damage

Wire sawing normal to the charge axis was used to expose sections of the damaged block for visual inspection. The number of cracks was counted in a quadrant from an aperture of 90° at 25-cm intervals radial from the blasthole. The lower quadrant opposite to the burden side was used for this crack count measure. The number of radial cracks or the number of cracks per arc length were compared to the MAE practical damage limit.

Practical Damage Limit

The practical damage limits were determined for the three concrete blocks using the MAE R_d approach (Table 7).

Table 7. Practical damage limit results for the three blocks tested

Block	R_d/r_h	MAE
1	30.0	0.57
2	29.8	0.57
3	30.8	0.58

Wave Attenuation Results

The radial strain measurements from all three blocks are listed in Table 8 and plotted in Figure 15. The seismic velocities of the waves converting strain to PPV are included in Table 8. The attenuation was similar for each experiment as shown by the plot and curve fit in Figure 15. The regression fit is exponential and was used to calculate radial limits at the uniaxial compressive strength (UCS) PPV limit from Persson et al. [1994], the experimental PPV seismic limit from Johnson [2010], and PPV values at the calculated MAE R_d limit. The equation fit is:

$$\varepsilon_{radial} = 0.00004x^{-2.078} \tag{12}$$

where ε_{radial} = the radial strain, and

x = distance (m).

Table 8. Strain measurements and PPV conversions for the three block experiments

Distance (m)	Block 1 strain	Block 1 PPV (m/sec)	Block 2 strain	Block 2 PPV (m/sec)	Block 3 strain	Block 3 PPV (m/sec)
0.15	0.0165	62.7	0.0195	76.635	nt	nt
0.23	nt*	nt	nt	nt	0.007	18.48
0.30	0.0066	25.08	0.0058	22.794	nt	nt
0.46	0.0026	9.88	0.003	11.79	0.002	5.28
0.61	0.0013	4.94	0.0007	2.751	nt	nt
0.69	nt	nt	nt	nt	0.001	2.64
0.91	nt	nt	nt	nt	0.0005	1.32
1.14	nt	nt	nt	nt	0.00025	0.66

*nt = not tested

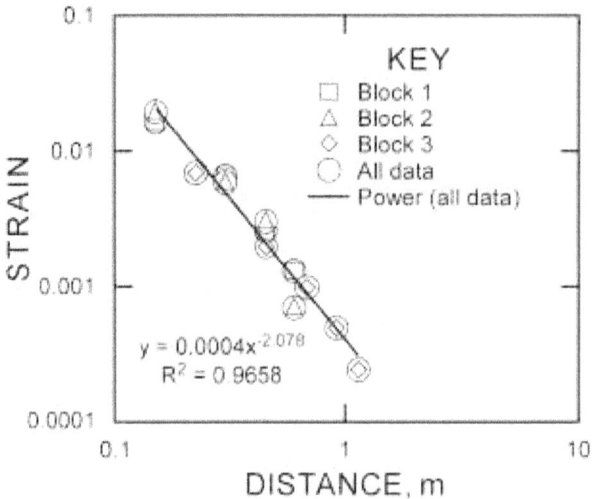

Figure 15. Plot of radial strain measurements for all three block experiments showing regression curve fit of all data.

Block 1 Damage Assessment

The damage measurement results are shown in three figures in this section. The damage measurements presented are shear wave seismic MVP (Figure 16), crosshole seismic (Figure 17), and radial crack count (Figure 19).

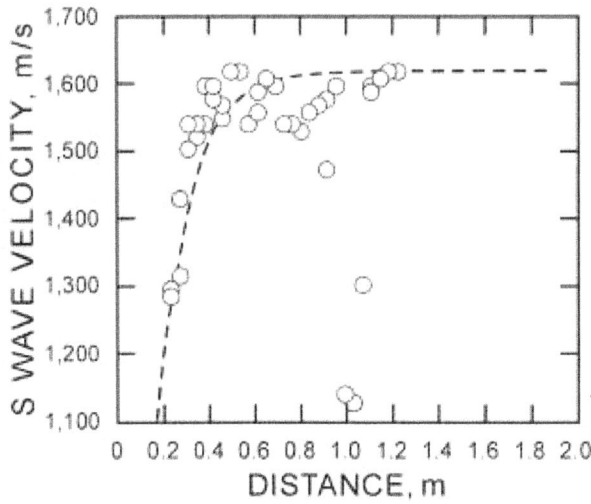

Figure 16. Block 1 MVP velocity vs. distance from blasthole.

The S-wave velocity data in Figure 16 shows damage closer than 0.4 m from the blasthole. There was a drop in velocity at about 1 m where a vertical crack was found. A curve was fit to the data to determine the distance at which the S-wave velocity reaches background levels for the undamaged block.

26

An exponential function was used to mathematically determine the limit of damage. The function was applied using the method of selected points to the data as shown in Figure 16. The function is described as:

$$y = a - e^{-bx}(a - k) \qquad (13)$$

where a = asymptote (m/sec),

b = decay,

x = radial distance (m), and

k = intercept at x = 0 (m/sec).

The selected fit for Equation 13 is a = 1,620 m/sec, b = 7, and k = 0 m/sec. The limit of 0.56-m distance is determined at 98% of the asymptote or 1,588 m/sec.

The seismic limit of 7.6 m/sec determined by Johnson [2010] for block 1 corresponds to 0.46-m radial distance using the seismic velocity of 3,800 m/sec and Equation 12. The crushing limit of 5.4 m/sec determined using the factor for the Persson et al. [1994] crushing limit for block 1 corresponds to 0.54-m radial distance using the seismic velocity of 3,800 m/sec and Equation 12.

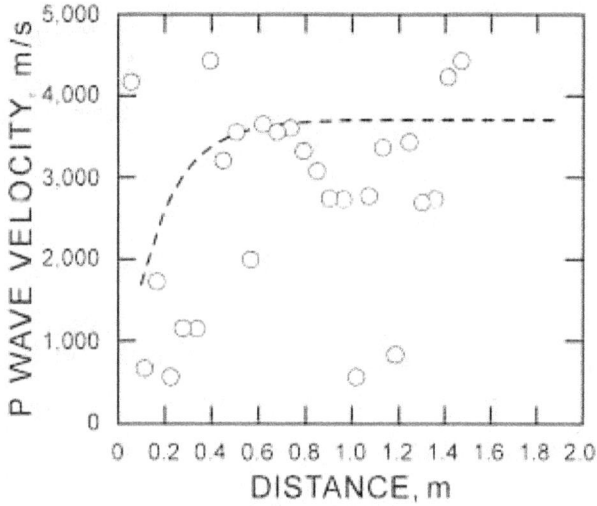

Figure 17. Block 1 postblast inspection hole damage assessment using the crosshole sonic P-wave velocity probes.

Crosshole P-wave sonic logging data were collected from inspection hole pairs spaced at 0.58 m. The results are plotted in Figure 17. The exponential function (Equation 13) was used to assess the limit of damage. The selected fit is a = 3,700 m/sec, b = 6, and k = 0 m/sec. The limit of 0.65-m distance is determined at 98% of the asymptote or 3,626 m/sec.

27

Radial cracks in block 1 were counted per unit arc length at radial intervals from the blasthole (Figure 18). The number of cracks and arc angles are listed in Table 9. There is a decrease in number of cracks per unit arc length with distance as shown in the plot in Figure 19.

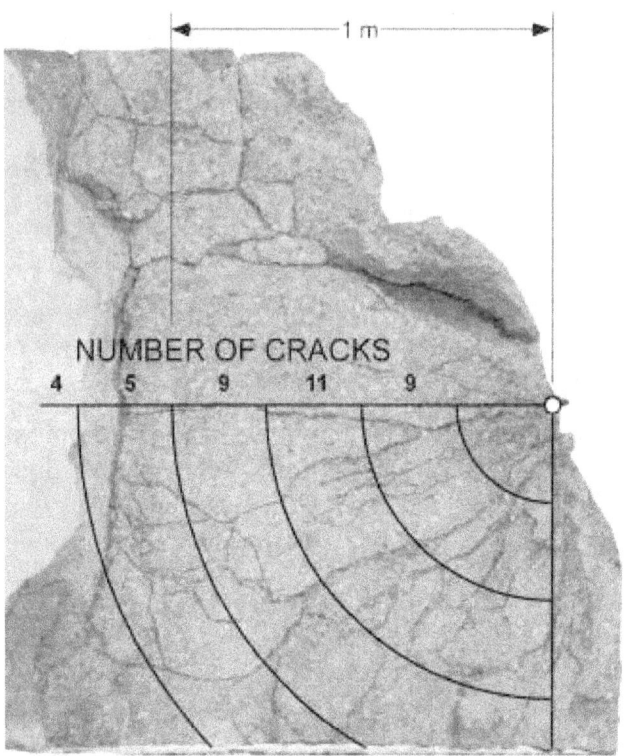

Figure 18. Block 1 photograph/quadrant overlay of postblast radial crack damage visible from wire saw cut.

Table 9. Block 1 number of radial cracks visible in wire saw cut

Quadrant	Radial distance (m)	Number of cracks	Aperture (degrees)	Cracks per m arc length
1	0.25	9	90	22.9
2	0.50	11	90	14.0
3	0.75	9	90	7.6
4	1.00	5	65	4.4
5	1.25	4	40	4.6

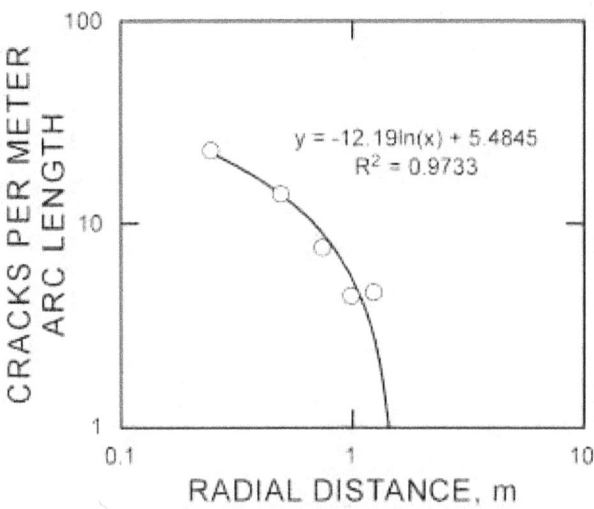

Figure 19. Block 1 postblast number of cracks counted with distance from the blasthole.

The number of cracks at the MAE R_d limit of 0.57 m using the regression equation in Figure 19 is 12.3 cracks per meter of arc length. The PPV as measured using strain at the MAE R_d limit is 4.9 m/sec.

Block 2 Damage Assessment

The damage measurement results are shown in the following figures. Damage measurements presented are crosshole seismic (Figure 20) and radial crack count (Figure 22).

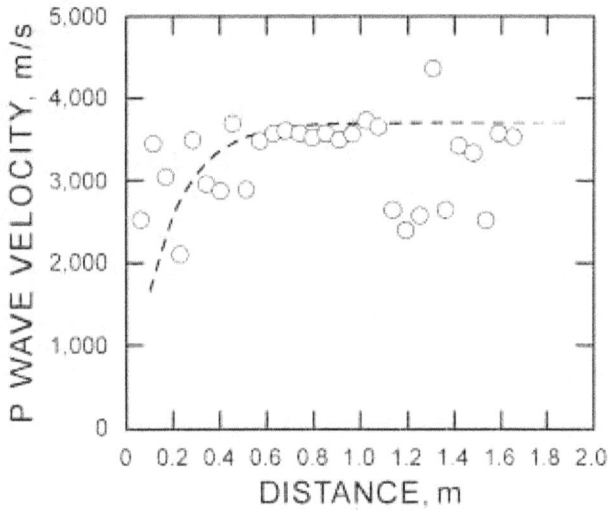

Figure 20. Block 2 inspection hole damage assessment using the crosshole sonic P-wave velocity probes.

Crosshole P-wave sonic logging data were collected from inspection hole pairs spaced at 0.58 m. The results are plotted in Figure 20. The exponential function was used to assess the limit of damage. The selected fit for Equation 13 is $a = 3,700$ m/sec, $b = 6$, and $k = 0$ m/sec. The limit of 0.65-m distance is determined at 98% of the asymptote or 3,626 m/sec.

The crushing limit of 5.2 m/sec that was determined using the factor for the Persson et al. [1994] crushing limit for block 2 corresponds to 0.56-m radial distance using the seismic velocity of 3,930 m/sec and Equation 12.

Radial cracks in block 2 were counted per unit arc length at radial intervals from the blasthole (Figure 21). The number of cracks and arc angles are listed in Table 10. There is a decrease in number of cracks per unit arc length with distance as shown in the plot in Figure 22.

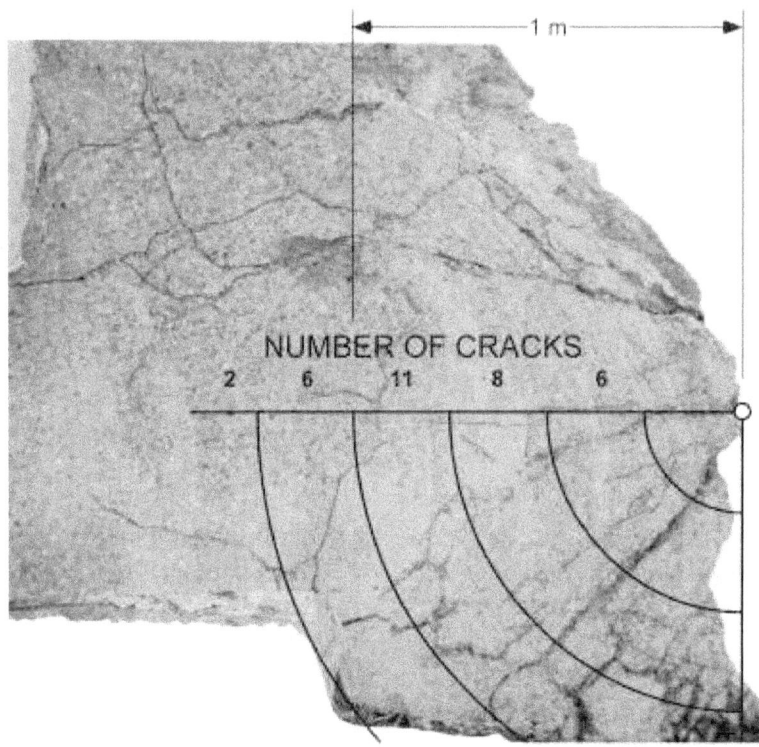

Figure 21. Block 2 photograph/quadrant overlay of postblast radial crack damage visible from wire saw cut.

Table 10. Block 2 number of radial cracks visible in wire saw cut

Distance (m)	Number of cracks	Aperture (degrees)	Cracks per m arc length
0.25	6	87	15.8
0.50	8	80	11.5
0.75	11	90	9.3
1.00	6	62	5.5
1.25	2	45	2.0

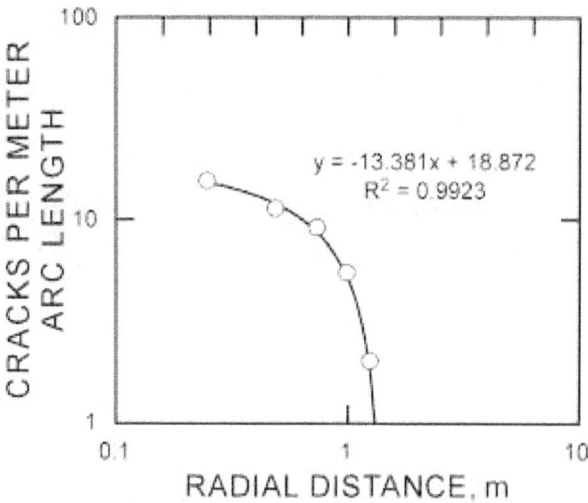

Figure 22. Block 2 number of cracks counted with distance from the blasthole.

The number of cracks at the MAE R_d limit of 0.57 m using the regression equation in Figure 22 is 11.2 cracks per meter of arc length. The PPV as measured using strain at the MAE R_d limit is 5.0 m/sec.

Block 3 Damage Assessment

The damage measurement results are shown in the following figures. Damage measurements presented are shear wave seismic MVP (Figure 23) and radial crack count (Figure 25).

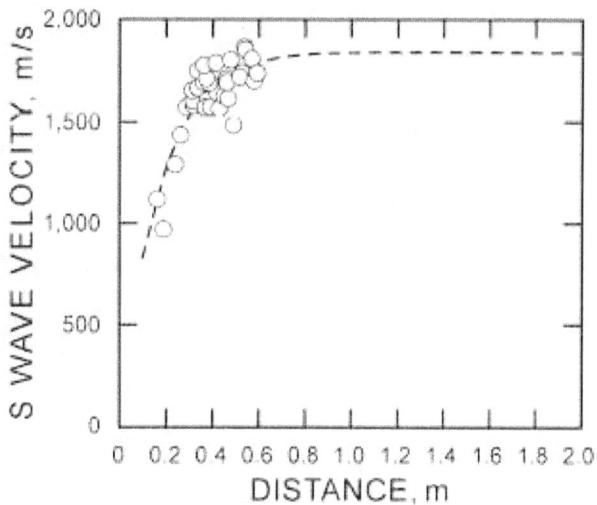

Figure 23. Block 3 postblast shear wave velocity as a function of distance from the blasthole with sensors oriented vertically.

Figure 23 shows the MVP results. The exponential function was used to assess the MVP measured damage limit. The selected fit as shown in Figure 23 using Equation 13 is $a = 1,850$ m/sec, $b = 6$, and $k = 0$ m/sec. The limit of 0.65-m distance is determined at 98% of the asymptote or 1,813 m/sec.

31

The seismic limit of 4.7 m/sec determined by Johnson for block 1 corresponds to 0.50-m radial distance using the seismic velocity of 2,640 m/sec and Equation 12. The crushing limit of 4.5 m/sec that was determined using the factor for the Persson et al. [1994] crushing limit for block 3 corresponds to 0.50-m radial distance using the seismic velocity of 2,640 m/sec and Equation 12.

Radial cracks in block 3 were counted per unit arc length at radial intervals from the blasthole (Figure 24). The number of cracks and arc angles are listed in Table 11. There is a decrease in number of cracks per unit arc length with distance as shown in the plot in Figure 25.

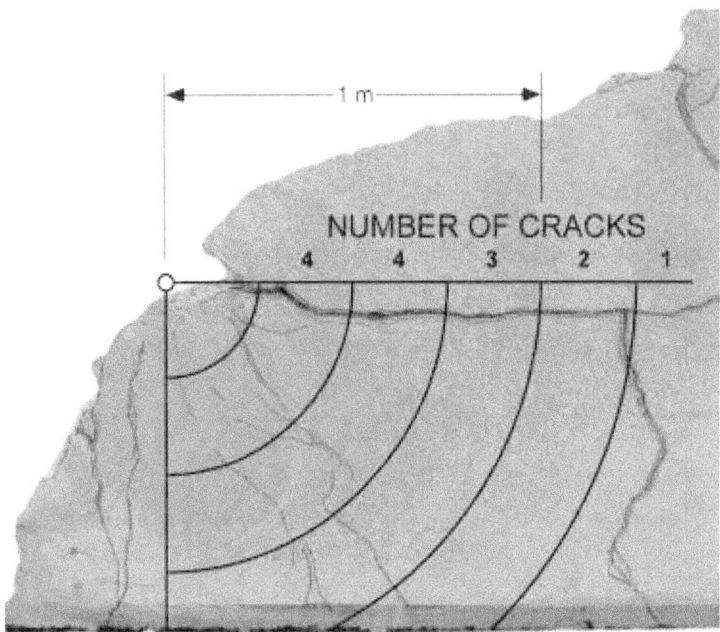

Figure 24. Block 3 photograph/quadrant overlay of postblast wire saw section near blasthole collar showing cracks.

Table 11. Block 3 number of radial cracks visible in wire saw cut

Distance (m)	Number of cracks	Aperture (degrees)	Cracks per m arc length
0.25	4	90	10.2
0.50	4	90	5.1
0.75	3	90	2.5
1.00	2	55	2.1
1.25	1	40	1.1

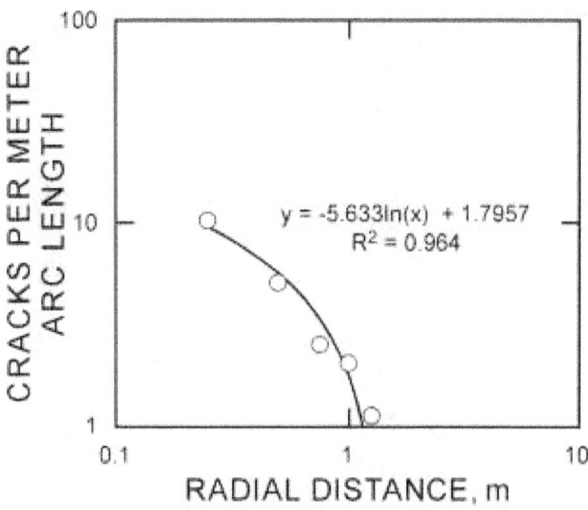

Figure 25. Block 3 postblast number of cracks vs. distance from blasthole.

The number of cracks at the MAE R_d limit of 0.57 m using the regression equation in Figure 25 is 4.9 cracks per meter of arc length. The PPV as measured using strain at the MAE R_d limit is 3.3 m/sec.

Discussion

Figure 26 provides a summary of the measured damage, predicted damage, and the calculated MAE R_d practical damage limit for each block tested. The measured damage using the MVP and the crosshole seismic methods correlates with the MAE R_d practical damage limit. Results are dependent on the percentage cutoff of the damage curve asymptote for each dataset. The measured limit is based on 98% of the asymptote and is slightly higher than the MAE R_d. The Persson et al. [1994] and Johnson [2010] PPV limit assessments for crushing and seismic limits are less than the MAE R_d practical damage limit but are within 80% of the MAE R_d value.

The number of radial cracks per meter of arc length estimated at the MAE R_d limit is 12.3, 11.2, and 4.9 for blocks 1, 2, and 3, respectively. The lower crack number for block 3 may indicate differences in parameters including block strength, block aggregate size, block density, explosive emulsion, charge length, and charge stemming. Blocks 1 and 2 had similar parameters and comparable crack results.

The measured PPV at the calculated MAE R_d practical damage limits for blocks 1, 2, and 3 are 4.9 m/sec, 5.0 m/sec, and 3.3 m/sec using the regression equation in Figure 15 and the seismic velocities.

The three block experiment results are data limited and preclude statistical analysis but provide a better understanding of the MAE R_d limit if used for blast design. When the MAE R_d limit is applied to a buffer hole design location, the MAE R_d limit would be expected to have radial cracks extending up to and beyond the limit, yet the primary damage expected by Persson et al. [1994] and by Johnson [2010] should be within the limit. The majority of damage as measured seismically using either the MVP or the crosshole techniques would occur up to the MAE R_d limit.

33

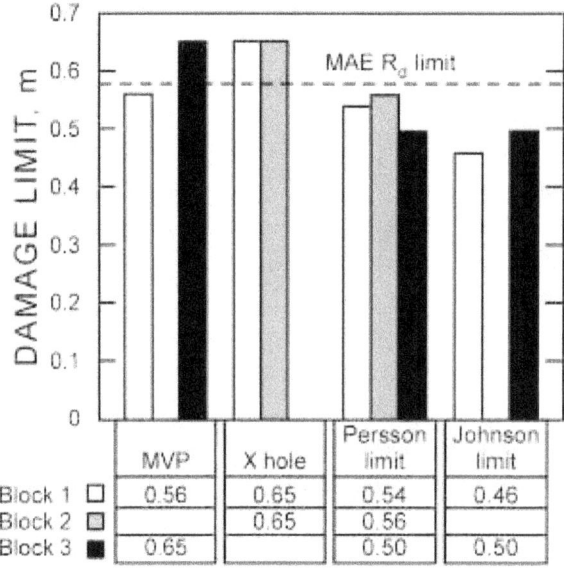

Figure 26. Summary of damage limit results of block experiments compared to MAE R_d.

	MVP	X hole	Persson limit	Johnson limit
Block 1 ☐	0.56	0.65	0.54	0.46
Block 2 ☐		0.65	0.56	
Block 3 ■	0.65		0.50	0.50

Buffer Hole Design Concept

The buffer hole concept is an adaptation of the practical damage limit for design. In the buffer hole design, the contour sector is determined by the buffer holes and not by the perimeter holes. The buffer concept was first published by Hustrulid and Johnson [2008]. The contour strip of rock is bounded on the inside by the buffer row of holes and on the outside by the perimeter (contour) row of holes. The detonation of the buffer row will produce damage in the contour sector. The idea is to design the buffer holes so that their associated damage radius extends to the desired drift perimeter. Figure 28 shows the case when the radius:

$$R_d = \text{contour row "burden"} \tag{14}$$

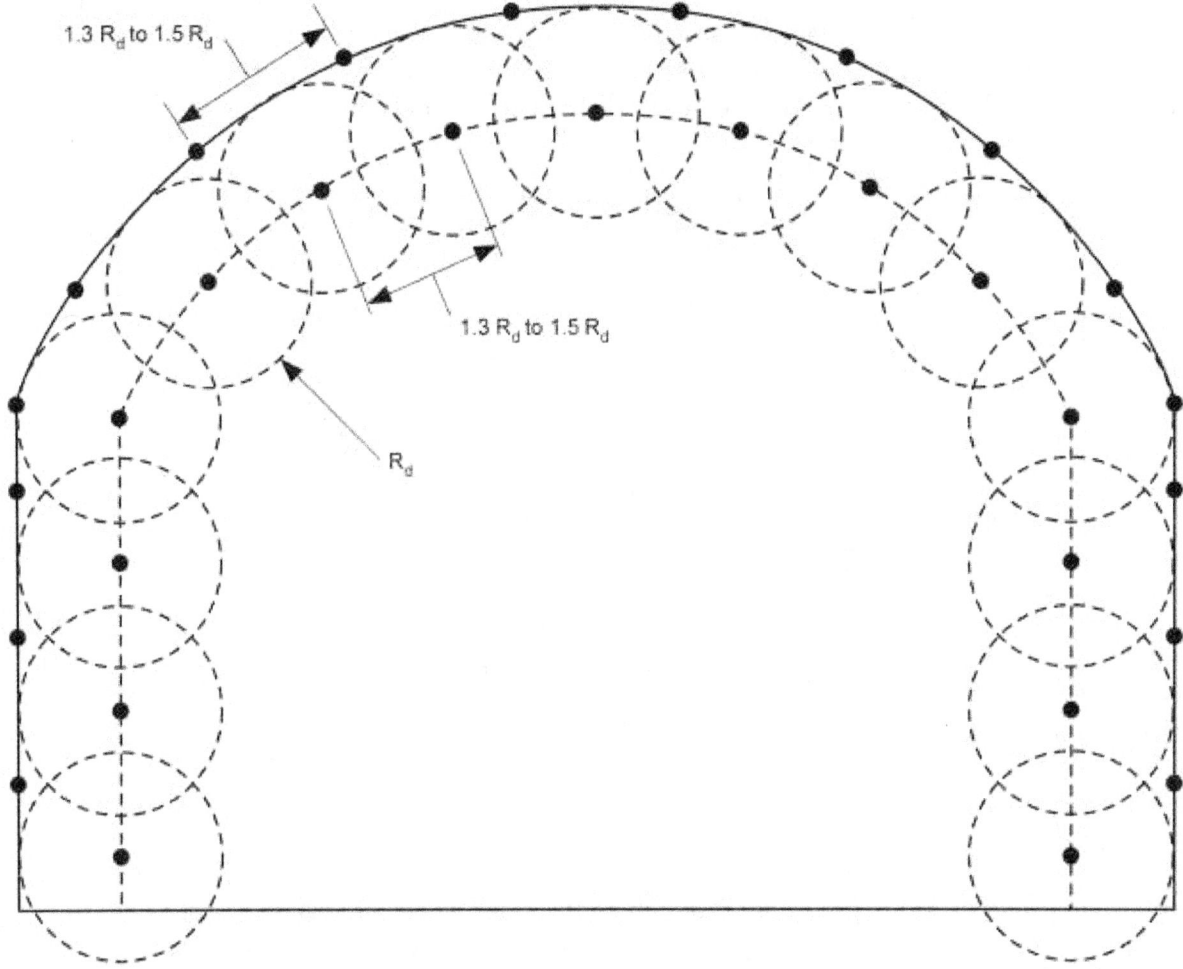

Figure 27. Buffer row hole locations, buffer hole practical damage circles, and perimeter holes at the cusp locations.

If this is the case, after the firing of the buffer holes, the amount of fresh/undamaged rock is only the small cusp of rock remaining between damage circles. With this in mind, the breaking demand on the perimeter holes is substantially reduced. This is a prime reason why the use of high-strength detonating cord often functions quite well as a perimeter control explosive because the primary function has become one of smoothing rather than primary breaking.

The key to the buffer row approach [Hustrulid and Johnson 2008] is the assignment of a "practical" radius of damage (R_d) to each blasthole/explosive combination being considered for use in the particular rock mass. The following steps are used after calculating the MAE R_d practical damage limit:

Step 1: Design the buffer row starting with buffer circles tangent to the abutment corners.
Step 2: Add the perimeter holes at the abutment corners and at the cusp locations.
Step 3: Design the lifters.
Step 4: Add the cut.
Step 5: Add stope B and C holes as required providing good energy coverage or based on powder factor experience.

35

Buffer hole spacing is suggested between 1.3 R_d and 1.5 R_d to provide area coverage of between 92.4% and 89.6% respectively. A plot of a wide range of buffer spacing factors and associated area coverages are shown in Figure 28. A high percentage area of coverage is advantageous for reducing the effort required for the perimeter charge. The 1.3 R_d and 1.5 R_d range is untested.

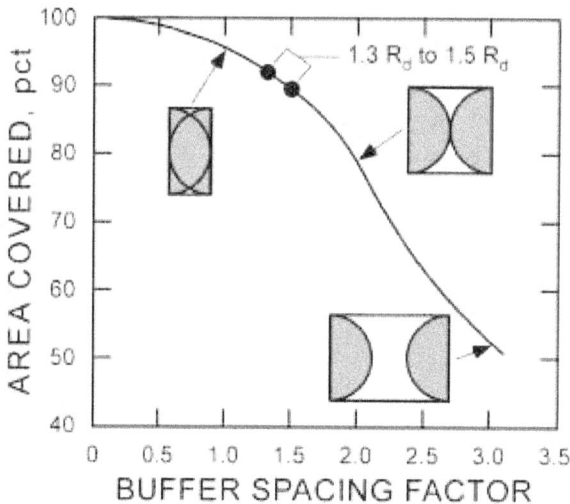

Figure 28. Range of buffer hole spacing conditions showing percentage of area covered by circles formed using the R_d damage radius.

Perimeter Charging

The buffer hole design procedure results in perimeter holes located at the cusps between buffer hole damage circles. Charging of the perimeter holes is decoupled to reduce the charge amount so as to crack the rock just sufficiently enough to trim the remaining rock. Sanden [1974] applied the force-equilibrium approach in developing a hole spacing (S) relationship for presplitting. The same perimeter spacing is suggested by Hustrulid and Johnson [2008] for contour blasting application using rock strength and explosion pressure using the equation

$$S = 2r_h \left(\frac{P_w + \sigma_t}{\sigma_t} \right) \tag{15}$$

where S = perimeter hole spacing (m),

r_h = blasthole radius (m),

P_w = explosion pressure exerted on the blasthole wall (MPa), and

σ_t = rock tensile strength (MPa).

36

If tensile strength is not known, a factor of, for example, 1/12 the compressive strength could be used. According to Hustrulid and Johnson [2008], P_w is designed to be less than the rock compressive strength to prevent rock crushing. However, the spacing result will likely be different than the buffer hole concept design spacing. Alternatively, with the spacing already determined by the buffer row concept design, the correct explosive amount could be determined by rearranging the Sanden [1974] equation where

$$P_w = \frac{S\sigma_t}{2r_h} - \sigma_t \tag{16}$$

The explosive and the calculated explosion wall pressure, using the pressure calculation described by Hustrulid and Johnson [2008], were chosen to match the pressure determined from Equation 16. Hustrulid and Johnson [2008] suggest the maximum wall pressure equal to the compressive strength of the rock to prevent crushing.

Discussion

In the buffer hole design concept the placement of the buffer holes determines the designed perimeter and the demand on the perimeter holes is substantially reduced. Perimeter charging options for the buffer design concept will require decoupling. Without perimeter hole decoupling, damage typical of an aggressive blast may result. Explosives manufacturers have products specifically suited for perimeter control; two examples are: (a) a detonation cord which comes in various charge concentrations and (b) emulsion-based trim cartridges or continuous charges. An alternative option is to use pumped emulsion or blown ANFO as a bottom charge. This reduces the overall energy in the perimeter hole. Another solution is to use ANFO fully coupled, in addition to tracing the ANFO with a detonation cord. The ANFO will not reach its velocity of detonation (VOD) potential, and the gas volume created from ANFO will split the rock similarly to a decoupled charge.

The use of detonators, boosters, or cartridges for initiation of the column charge is not considered in the buffer design. The length of the blastholes and the resulting length of the blast round are not considered in the buffer design. The design considers the buffer and perimeter holes to be drilled parallel to each other. Rock structure is not considered in the buffer row concept design, even though the rock structure can affect the blast outcome. Singh and Narendrula [2007] have done considerable research on the influence of rock structure. Research indicates that blasthole spacing should be less than the joint spacing because radial cracks will likely arrest at a joint surface. Hustrulid [1999a] indicates that closer joint spacing requires more blastholes of smaller diameter.

Analysis of Successful Perimeter Control Designs

Introduction

Successful controlled blast designs provide as-built results that are equivalent to as-designed results. The perimeter is controlled and typically results in half-barrel remnants from the perimeter holes indicating no overbreak and only minimal fracturing into the perimeter. Five successful perimeter control designs were chosen to show the relevance of the buffer row concept and any differences between both design concepts. The following sections provide a comparison of the buffer hole design concept to the five successful designs including a comparison of buffer hole placement, perimeter hole spacing, and hole charging.

Example of a Successful String-Loading Perimeter Control Design

Decoupling through the process of string-loading bulk emulsion in the perimeter holes is thought to be a very appealing alternative which should be considered by U.S. mining companies. Although not available in the United States at the time of this writing, string loading is a common method for perimeter control elsewhere in the world. This technique offers a relatively simple means for applying perimeter control for use in production holes and is desirable for wet conditions, thereby reducing the number of types of explosives in the round to just one. The variable speed charging hose retraction rate offered by the string-loading equipment allows the miner to adjust the perimeter decoupling ratio. Figure 29 illustrates the string-loading process.

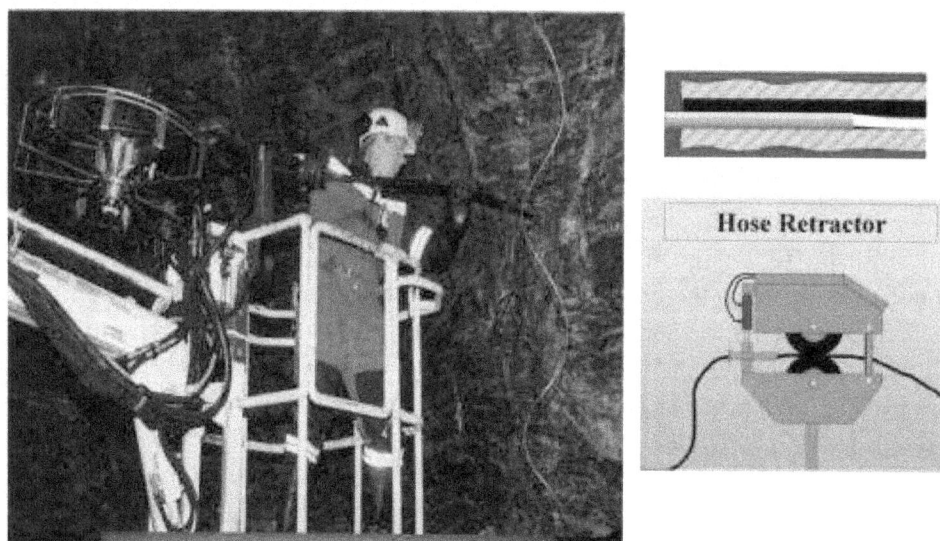

Figure 29. Photograph and diagrams of string-loading bulk emulsion using constant pumping and variable rate extraction of the injection hose [Fauske 2003; Hustrulid 2008].

A successful controlled blast design using string loading is currently being applied at a mine in Australia (see Figure 30). This design will serve as the basis for analysis using the buffer row concept because the position of the buffer row is parallel to the perimeter and approximately at the correct damage distance from the perimeter. This is considered a successful design because the as-designed limit is equivalent to the as-drilled limit and the as-built limit. Damage beyond the as-built limit is subjective because no measure of radial cracks was made. Overbreak has been minimized and the perimeter is defined by the perimeter blasthole half-barrels.

The basis used for the design, especially the buffer row distance from the perimeter, is uncertain. It may in fact be based on a standard empirical-based design or a special design from the mine's expert consultant. This design was selected as the one that most closely follows the buffer row design.

The authors of this report visited the Australian mine site and collected geotechnical and design data.

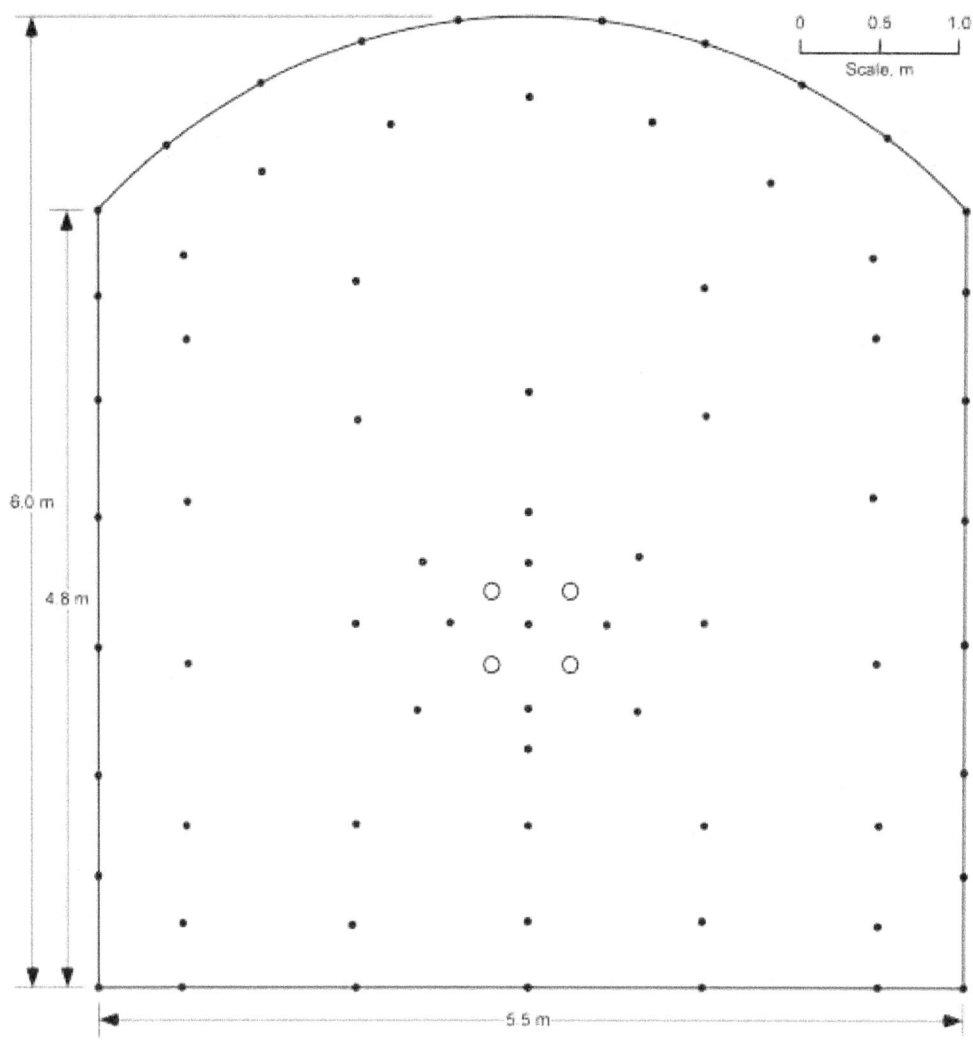

Figure 30. Example showing drill hole locations of a successful blast design in Australia that uses string-loaded emulsion.

Explosive Properties

The round was drilled using a computer-controlled drill jumbo. The round was charged using site-sensitized emulsion. The explosive properties include energy at 3.1 MJ/kg (740 kcal/kg), gas volume at about 950 L/kg, density at 0.85 g/cm^3, VOD equal to 4,300 m/s, and relative weight strength (RWS) or s_{ANFO} equal to 0.84. The buffer holes were fully charged and the perimeter holes were string loaded to 50% of the hole cross-sectional area (0.034 m in diameter). The adiabatic constant γ is assumed to be 3.0.

Drift Geometry

The drift geometry is 5.5 m wide, 4.8 m to the abutment corners, and 6 m to the crown. Blasthole length was 6 m and the hole diameters were 48 mm. The buffer row R_d was 0.54 m. A buffer row is prominent with a spacing of 0.85 m (1.57 R_d). The perimeter row spacing was 0.65 m (0.2 R_d).

40

Rock Properties

The rock type is monzonite with a density of 2.8 g/cm^3 and a Poisson's ratio of 0.28. The rock friction angle is 45°. The compressive strength is 150 MPa and the tensile strength is 22 MPa from Brazilian tests.

Blast Damage Calculations

The calculated MAE R_d practical damage limit for the fully coupled buffer holes is 0.54 m or 22.5 blasthole radius.

Discussion

Table 12 compares the calculations of the buffer design approach to the successful design. Being a successful design implies that there is no improvement needed. However, it is useful to compare the successful design to provide validation to the buffer design approach. The successful design shows several important relationships using the applied R_d practical damage radius. The successful design perimeter burden or buffer hole R_d is equal to the MAE calculated R_d of 0.54 m.

The buffer hole spacing measured on the design is 0.85 m or 1.57 times the designed R_d of 0.54 m and is slightly larger than the suggested buffer hole spacing range of 1.3R_d to 1.5R_d. The perimeter hole spacing is 0.65 m and is less than the buffer hole spacing of 0.85 m.

Table 12. Buffer row design concept parameters and damage compared to successful Australian design

Design	R_d (m)	Buffer spacing	Perimeter spacing	Sanden perimeter P_w (MPa)
MAE	0.54	1.3 R_d to 1.5 R_d	1.3 R_d to 1.5 R_d	300 to 349
Successful design	0.54	1.57 R_d	1.2 R_d	275 (598 covolume wall pressure)

Spacing of the perimeter holes at the cusps, which is part of the buffer row design concept, occurs for 9 of the 21 perimeter holes in the successful design. If the buffer design concept was applied (buffer holes alternate with perimeter holes), the result would be a larger spacing of perimeter holes and less perimeter holes than used in the successful design.

The Sanden [1974] perimeter charge wall pressure equation results are less than the decoupled, string-loaded wall pressure of 598 MPa of the successful design [Hustrulid 2010]. The decoupled pressure calculation is shown in Table 20 in the Appendix. The Sanden [1974] calculated pressures needed for the various perimeter spacings all exceeded the compressive strength of 150 MPa.

Example of a Successful Bottom Charge Perimeter Control Design

This successful development drift design is used at a block cave operation in the United States.

Explosive Properties

The blastholes were charged with ANFO. A detonator and booster were used for initiation. For perimeter control, ANFO was used for the back perimeter holes by charging the bottom third of the hole and leaving the upper two thirds of the hole empty. The collar was typically plugged to provide an air deck between the collar and the bottom charge. The result was a decrease in the overall explosion pressure over the uncharged length of the hole, even though the bottom third was fully coupled. The perimeter charge explosion pressure calculation requires an assumption that the bottom charge explosion pressure is reduced over the uncharged hole length. The fully coupled bottom charge volume is distributed along the entire hole length as:

$$\pi r_{charge}^2 L_{charge} = \pi r_{decoupled}^2 L_{hole} \tag{17}$$

where r_{charge} = bottom charge radius (m),

L_{charge} = bottom charge length (m),

$r_{decoupled}$ = assumed charge radius for decoupling calculation (m), and

L_{hole} = assumed charge length for decoupling calculation = hole length (m).

The equation is solved for $r_{decoupled}$ and a decoupled explosion pressure is calculated (Appendix Table 21). In the case for the successful design bottom charge, with the average hole length of 4.4 m and a bottom charged length of 1.5 m, the assumed decoupled charge diameter is 0.014 m.

Drift Geometry

The drift design (Figure 31) is nominally 4.28 m x 4.27 m in cross section with an arched roof and an abutment height of 2.1 m. A line of buffer holes parallels the perimeter holes defining a perimeter burden of 0.76 m. Blastholes were 0.048 m in diameter and 4.4 m long. The perimeter burden (buffer hole R_d) is 0.73 m and the buffer hole spacing is 0.8 m or 1.1 R_d. The perimeter hole spacing is 0.73 m (1.0 R_d).

Rock Properties

The mine geology consists of quartz vein stock works. The rock type was primarily porphyritic with a compressive strength of 77 MPa, a density of 2.5 kg/m^3 and a Poisson's ratio of 0.22. The rock mass quality was determined to have a Rock Mass Rating (RMR) of 48.

Blast Damage Calculations

The calculated MAE R_d practical damage limit for the fully coupled buffer holes is 0.68 m or 28.3 blasthole radius.

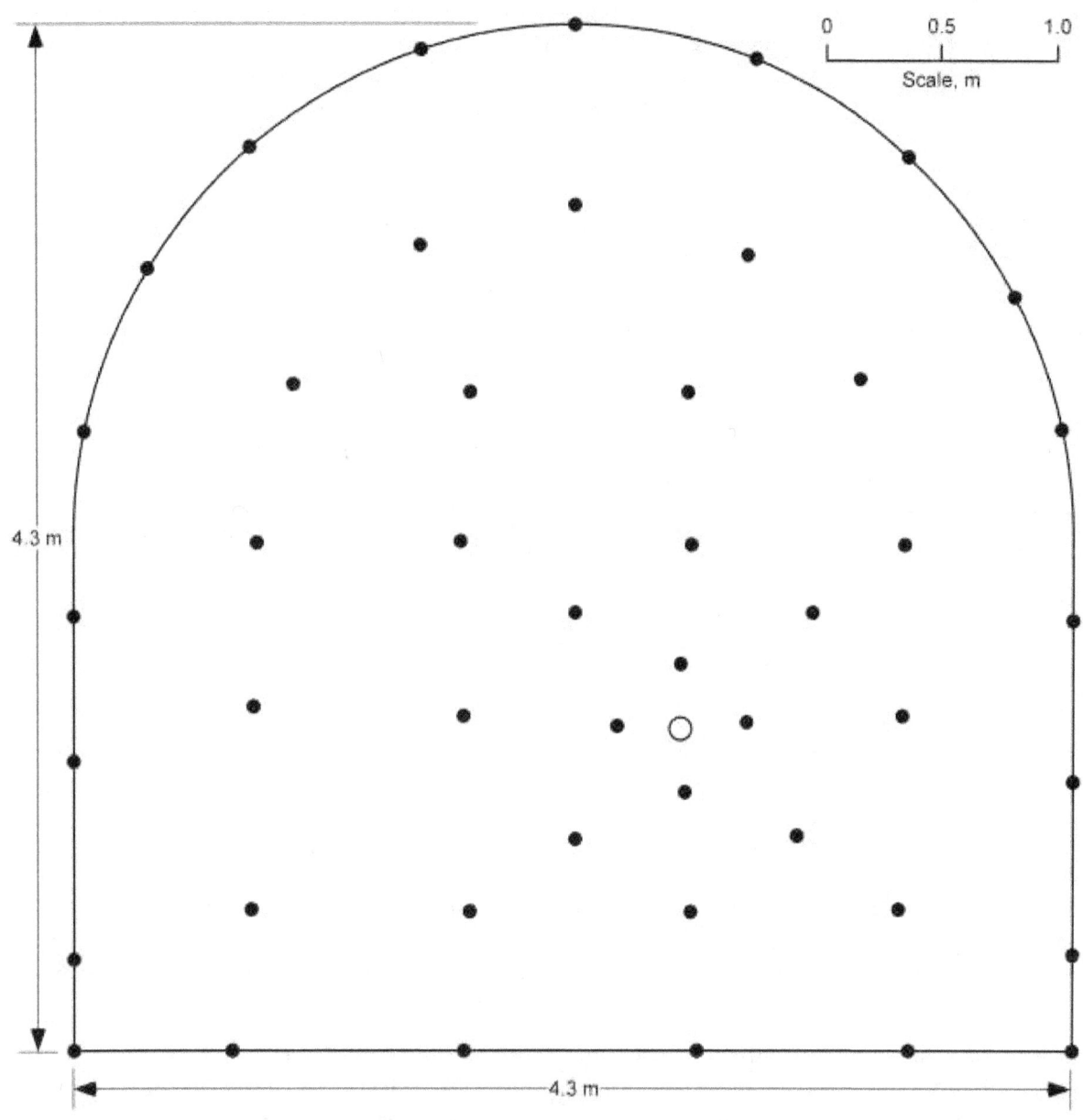

Figure 31. Example of a successful blast design in the United States with bottom-charged perimeter holes.

Discussion

Table 13 compares the buffer design approach calculations to the successful design. The successful mine design employs a common perimeter control practice of bottom charging the perimeter holes to reduce the explosion energy and in turn reducing perimeter damage. Though not as effective as a full-length decoupled charge, the bottom charging method does reduce damage compared to fully coupled charging and can be considered a successful blast design. Perimeter damage along the fully coupled section (bottom charge) of the perimeter holes is expected to have greater damage than the air-decked section.

The successful design buffer hole locations compared well with the damage model. The successful perimeter hole spacing is less than what would be expected for the buffer design concept of 1.3 R_d to 1.5 R_d. However, the successful perimeter spacing of 1.0 R_d is nearly equivalent to the buffer spacing of 1.1 R_d for the successful design indicating perimeter holes are at the cusps. Equivalent buffer and perimeter spacing is a requirement for the buffer design concept.

The successful design provides additional insight into possible adjustments for the buffer row design concept. It might be worthwhile to try a buffer hole spacing less than the conceptual range of 1.3 R_d to 1.5 R_d. The successful perimeter hole spacing would then align with the new buffer hole cusp locations. The actual decoupled pressure calculation of 56 MPa is less than the required calculated pressures by Sanden [1974]. The actual decoupled pressure calculation is shown in Table 21 in the Appendix.

Table 13. Buffer row design concept parameters and damage compared to successful U.S. design

Design	R_d (m)	Buffer spacing	Perimeter spacing	Sanden perimeter P_w (MPa)
MAE	0.68	1.3 R_d to 1.5 R_d	1.3 R_d to 1.5 R_d	112 to 130
Successful design	0.73	1.1 R_d	1 R_d	91 (56 covolume wall pressure)

Example of a Successful Swedish Decoupled Cartridge Perimeter Control Design

This design example is an underground zinc/silver operation. The mine uses cut and fill stoping techniques in steep-dipping narrow veins in rock that is primarily limestone [Norling and Nord 2006]. Information for this analysis is based on design information from Norling and Nord [2006] and personal communication from Marklund [2011].

The mine had previously used contract miners for drift driving. There was a concern about overbreak problems and the apparent poor rock quality after blasting. A new blast design was implemented using in-house resources for both drilling and blasting. The new blast design is shown in Figure 32. The design shows the use of perimeter control by using: (1) close-spaced perimeter holes and (2) a buffer row parallel to the perimeter row. A two-relief hole burn cut is used with stoping B holes on each side of the burn cut, stope C holes above the burn cut, knee holes below the burn cut, and lifters to define the floor.

Explosive Properties

The properties of the explosives used for this blast design are shown in Table 14. Note that, with the exception of ANFO, all of the charges are decoupled.

The published relative weight strengths of the explosives are shown in Table 14. The s_{ANFO} values were also calculated from the gas volume and energy of the explosives as provided by the mine. Properties for the Emulit 22 gas volume were not available from the mine. The following Swedish equation is used to calculate the relative weight strength with respect to a base explosive:

$$s = \frac{5}{6}\frac{Q}{Q_0} + \frac{1}{6}\frac{V}{V_0} \tag{18}$$

where s = Relative weight strength,

Q = Explosive energy (MJ/kg),

Q_0 = Base explosive energy (MJ/kg),

V = Explosive gas volume (m³/kg), and

V_0 = Base explosive (ANFO) (m³/kg).

In this example ANFO has been used as the base explosive. The referenced weight strengths compared well with the calculated values.

Table 14. Successful Swedish controlled blast design explosive properties

Hole	Type	Diameter (mm)	Density	s_{ANFO}, published weight strength	*VOD* (km/sec)	*Q* (MJ/kg)	*V* (m³/kg)	s_{ANFO}, calculated weight strength
Perimeter	Gurit 17	17	1,000	0.85	2.4	3.4	.930	0.87
Buffer	Emulit 22	22	1,130	nd*	5	2.4	1.12	0.69
Stope and cut	ANFO	48	850	1.0	2.2	4.0	.970	1.0
Lifter	Dynamex 32	32	1,450	1.13	4.5	4.5	.890	1.09

Sources: Norling and Nord [2006], Persson et al. [1994], Holmberg [1992], and Hustrulid and Johnson [2008].
*nd = not determined

Geometry

The drift dimensions are 5 m wide, 4.9 m to the abutment corners, and 6 m in overall height. All holes are 4 m in length and 0.048 m in diameter. The perimeter burden (buffer hole R_d) is 0.5 m, and the buffer hole spacing ranges from 0.7 m to 1.0 m. The perimeter hole spacing is 0.7 m.

Rock Properties

The rock type is limestone in generally good ground based on the RMR of 75 or higher. Table 15 lists some of the important rock properties [Markland 2011].

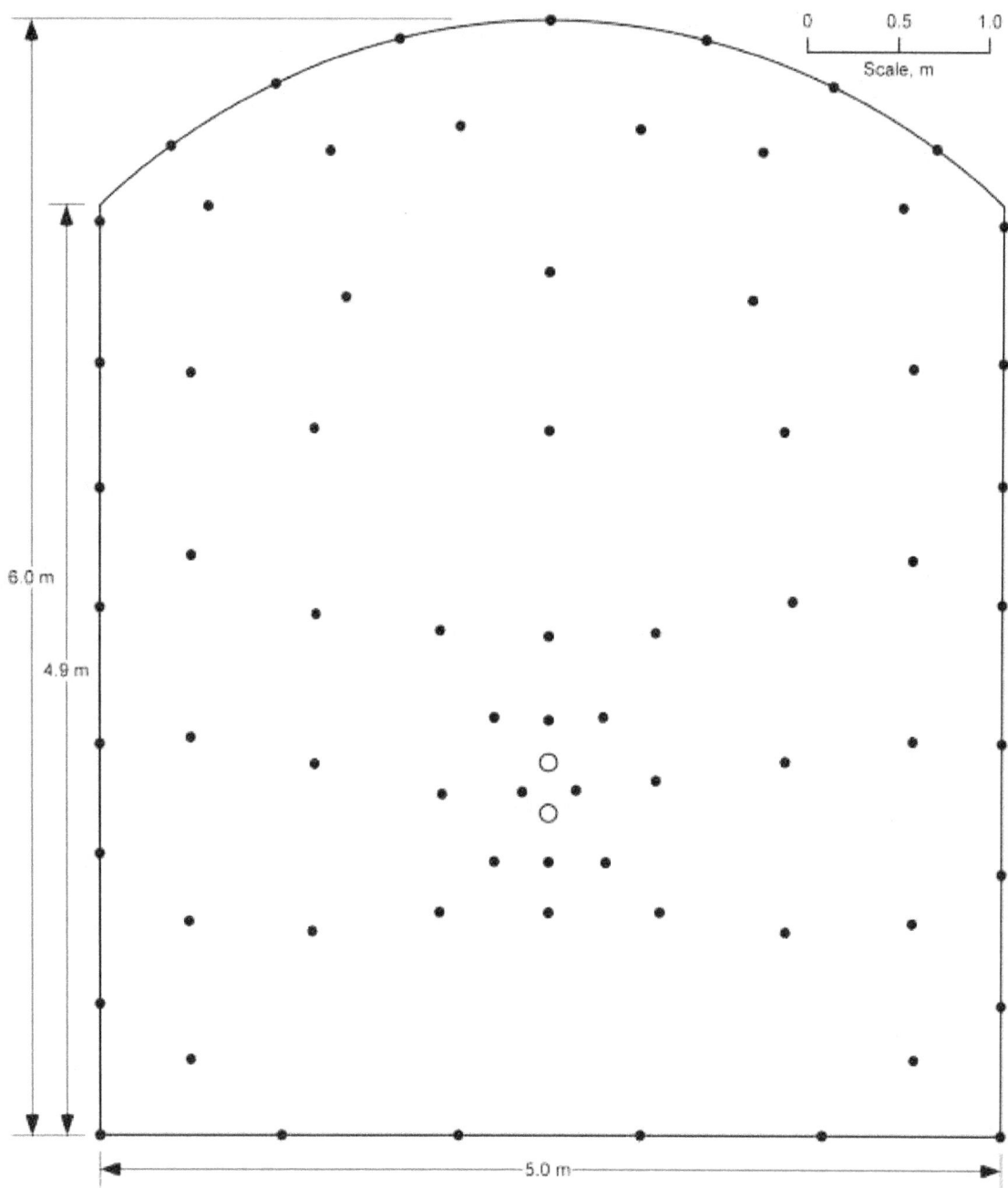

Figure 32. Example of the successful blast design in Sweden with decoupled perimeter cartridges.

Table 15. Properties of rock at the example mine

Property	Value
Rock type	Limestone
RMR	>75
Modulus of elasticity	60 GPa
Poisson's ratio	0.12
UCS	100 MPa
Density	2,700 kg/m^3
Sonic velocity	4,860 m/sec
Friction angle	Unknown (45° assumed)

Blast Damage Calculations

The calculated MAE R_d practical damage limit for the decoupled buffer holes is 0.30 m or 12.5 blasthole radius. The MAE calculation presented in this report does not account for decoupling. The MAE result was multiplied by the decoupling ratio as described by Hustrulid [2010] to best estimate the decoupled MAE R_d value.

Discussion

The buffer design approach calculations are compared to the successful design in Table 16. The MAE damage calculation for Emulit 22 for the buffer row R_d was 0.30 m and less than the successful design R_d of 0.5 m. The successful design's 0.7-m perimeter spacing is correct for the buffer row design concept range of 1.3 R_d to 1.5 R_d. The successful design's back buffer hole spacing also fell within the 1.3 R_d to 1.5 R_d design concept range. The rib buffer spacing was greater than the design concept range. Perimeter charge wall pressure was calculated to be 33 MPa. The Sanden equation results were higher. The decoupled pressure calculation is shown in the Appendix in Table 22.

Table 16. Buffer row design concept parameters and damage compared to successful Swedish design

Design	R_d (m)	R_d/r_h	Buffer spacing	Perimeter spacing	Sanden Perimeter P_w (MPa)
MAE	0.3	12.5	1.3 R_d to 1.5 R_d	1.3 R_d to 1.5 R_d	59 to 70
Successful design	0.50	22.2	1.4 R_d to 2.0 R_d	1.4 R_d	113 (33 covolume wall pressure)

Example of a Successful Canadian Controlled Blast Design

The successful Canadian design example is from an underground nickel mine using cut-and-fill and vertical block mining methods [Marshall et al. 1983]. This successful development controlled blast design has been described by Sutherland [1989] and Cudmore [2001]. The design utilized a buffer row approach with careful perimeter blasting using an Orica Powersplit perimeter control explosive. The perimeter and buffer hole placements are shown in Figure 33.

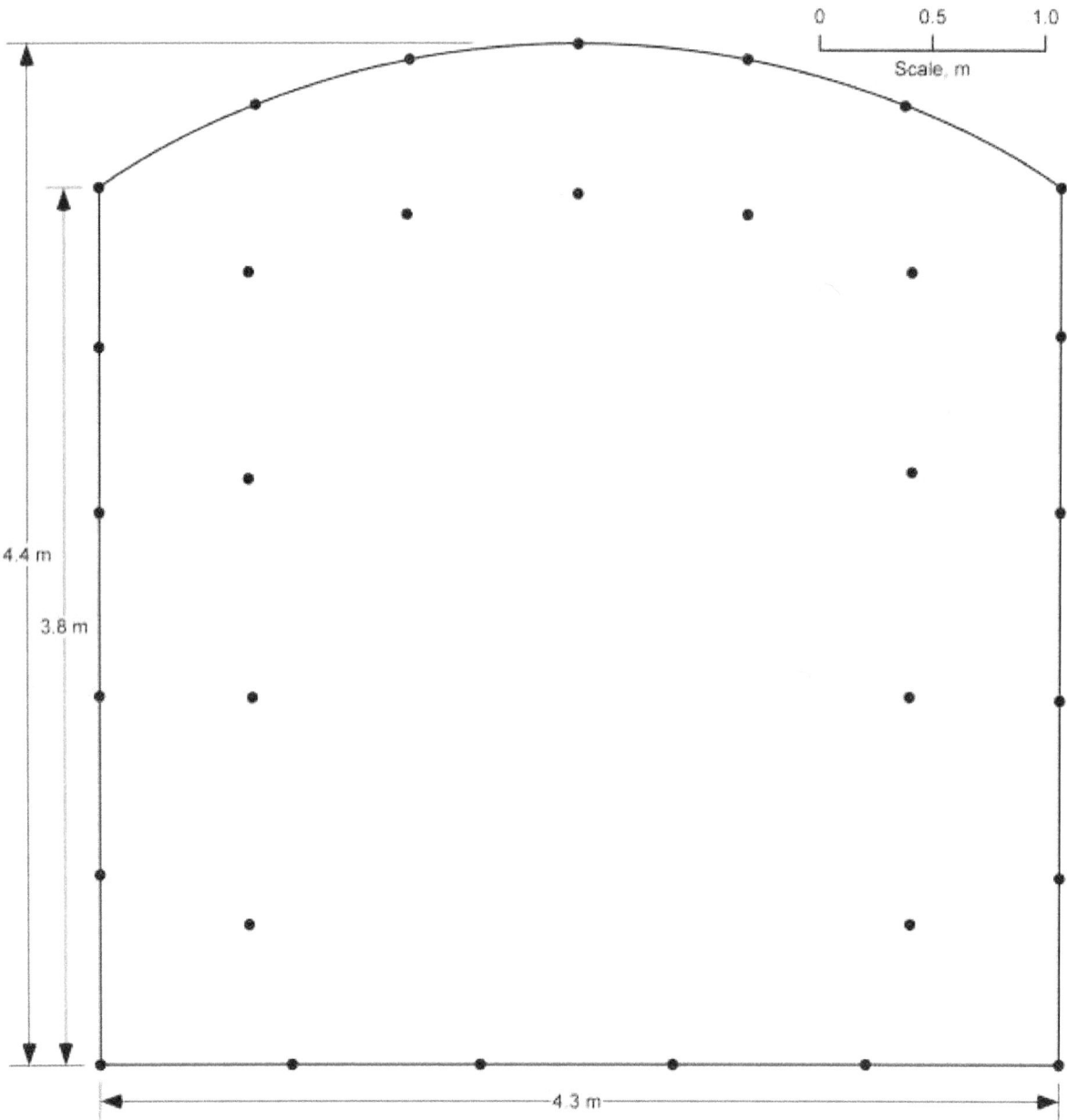

Figure 33. Example of a successful blast design in Canada with decoupled perimeter cartridges (shown are only the locations of the buffer, perimeter, and lifter holes).

Explosive Properties

The perimeter control explosive that proved most effective for the successful Canadian design was the 22-mm-diameter, continuous-packaged Orica Powersplit slurry product. The buffer and production holes were charged with Amex™ ANFO. The explosive properties are listed in Table 17.

Table 17. Explosives used for Canadian successful design

Explosive	Density (kg/m³)	Explosive diameter (m)	Published VOD (km/sec)	RWS
Orica Amex	1,000	0.048	3.3	1.1
Orica Senatel Powersplit (traced with 10 g/m det cord)	1,300	0.022	7	1.09

Geometry

According to Sutherland [1989], the perimeter hole burden and spacing were based on the hole diameter where $k = 15$ to 16 and the burden was 0.8 of the spacing as described in the Modified Ash Energy (MAE) Approach section. The development drift dimensions were 4.3 m wide, 3.8 m to the abutment height, and 4.4 m in total height. The blastholes were 45 mm in diameter and 3.6 m in length. The perimeter burden (buffer hole R_d) was 0.66 m. The buffer hole spacing was 0.95 m for the rib buffer holes and 0.71 m for the back buffer holes. Perimeter hole spacing was 0.8 for the ribs and 0.76 m for the back.

Rock Properties

The rock was schistose gneiss with assumed rock properties of 150 MPa compressive strength, 0.25 Poisson's ratio, and a 45° friction angle.

Blast Damage Calculations

The calculated MAE R_d practical damage limit for the fully coupled buffer holes is 0.62 m or 27.6 blasthole radius.

Discussion

The buffer design approach calculations are compared to the successful design in Table 18. The successful buffer row R_d was comparable to the MAE results. The buffer spacing of 1.1 R_d to 1.4 R_d was also comparable to the suggested buffer design spacing of 1.3 R_d to 1.5R_d. Perimeter spacing was slightly less than the suggested buffer design spacing. The Sanden [1974] perimeter explosion pressure for the successful design was comparable to the Sanden calculated pressures for the MAE buffer design approach calculations. The actual decoupled perimeter hole wall pressure was calculated to be 612 MPa. This pressure seems high and is the result of a higher VOD and density values for the traced detonation cord combined with the Senatel emulsion explosive. The decoupled pressure calculation is shown in the Appendix in Table 23.

Table 18. Buffer row design concept parameters and damage compared to successful Canadian design

Design	R_d (m)	Buffer spacing	Perimeter spacing	Sanden Perimeter P_w (MPa)
MAE	0.62	1.3 R_d to 1.5 R_d	1.3 R_d to 1.5 R_d	211 to 245
Successful design	0.66	1.1 R_d to 1.4R_d	1.2 R_d	208 (612 covolume wall pressure)

Example of a Successful Spanish Railway Tunnel Construction Controlled Blast Design

This railway tunnel design is the initial upper cut of the tunnel. The site was visited by the authors of this paper in 2009, and geotechnical and design data were collected. As seen in the upper cut design in Figure 34, the buffer holes are at a constant distance from the perimeter and are equally spaced.

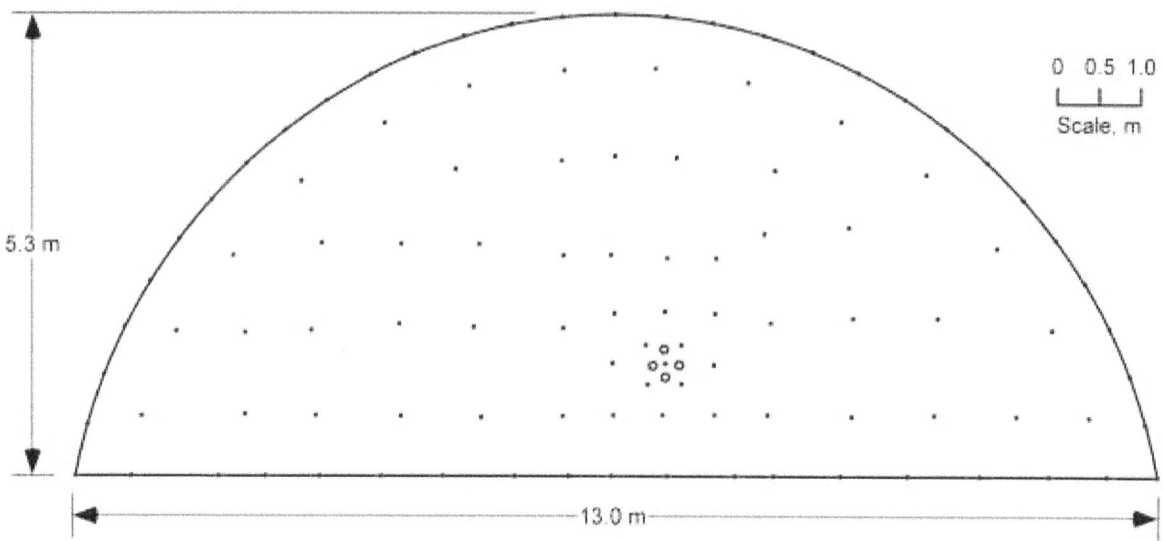

Figure 34. Example of the successful railway tunnel blast design in Spain.

Explosive Properties

The perimeter holes were bottom charged with two sticks of a cartridge explosive and a 100-gram/m detonation cord with an assumed VOD of 7 km/sec. For the explosion pressure calculation, the diameter of the contained PETN in the detonation cord was determined to be 0.0095 m assuming a density of 1,400 kg/m³. The production and buffer holes were charged with a gelatin nitroglycerin-based explosive, Goma 2 E-C, widely used for industrial applications in Spain. The bottom 1.2 m of the holes was charged with 40-mm-diameter cartridges, and the remaining 0.8-m charged length was loaded with 32-mm cartridges. The similar properties of the Orica Powerfrac were used for the buffer damage model calculations.

Geometry

The tunnel heading was 13 m wide and 5.34 m high. The blastholes were 3 m long and 45 mm in diameter. The perimeter burden (buffer row R_d) was 0.57 m. The buffer row spacing was 1.17 m. The perimeter row spacing was 0.62 m.

Rock Properties

The rock type was limestone with RMR values ranging from 35 to 60. The compressive strength ranged from 25 MPa to 60 MPa. The friction angle ranged from 28° to 39°. Poisson's ratio was assumed to be 0.25. Rock density was assumed to be 2.65 g/cm^3.

Blast Damage Calculations

The calculated MAE R_d practical damage limit for the fully coupled buffer holes was 0.67 m or 29.8 blasthole radius.

Discussion

The buffer design approach calculations are compared to the successful design in Table 19. The successful tunnel design provides additional insight for comparison to the buffer row design approach. The design had a distinct buffer row with a consistent distance R_d of 0.57 m to the perimeter. The MAE calculated R_d was greater than the successful design R_d.

The successful buffer hole spacing of 2.1 R_d was higher than the concept design suggested of 1.3 R_d to 1.5 R_d.

The successful design required closer perimeter spacing than suggested by the concept design. The calculated Sanden [1974] perimeter wall pressure P_w for splitting was 65 MPa and less than the actual wall pressure of 84 MPa. The MAE calculated splitting pressure was reasonably close to the pressure calculated for the successful design perimeter charge. The decoupled pressure calculation is shown in the Appendix in Table 24.

Table 19. Buffer row design concept parameters and damage compared to successful tunnel design

Design	R_d (m)	Buffer spacing	Perimeter spacing	Sanden perimeter P_w (MPa)
MAE	0.67	1.3 R_d to 1.5 R_d	1.3 R_d to 1.5 R_d	91 to 107
Successful design	0.57	2.1 R_d	1.1 R_d	65 (84 covolume wall pressure)

Discussion

The average buffer row R_d ratio (R_d/r_h) for the successful designs was 24.4. This is only slightly less than the MAE R_d approach base value of 25. In most of the comparisons the damage model R_d values correlate with the successful design R_d values. The buffer hole R_d values that were appreciably different were the successful Swedish and Spanish designs. Discrepancies in the buffer row concept design include the slight differences in the buffer hole spacing and consistently fewer perimeter holes. The Sanden calculations for perimeter hole pressure are interesting in that two of the successful designs had much higher pressures than required for splitting between perimeter holes. Conversely, three of the successful designs had lower pressures than suggested by Sanden [1974], although perimeter smoothing was successful. The successful low perimeter hole wall pressures indicated that the requirement of splitting between perimeter holes is unnecessary and only cusp removal or local perimeter smoothing was required.

Design Guidance

Some guidance is suggested for the user applying the buffer row design approach. These guidance points are based on the data and analysis presented in this report. Guidance points relating to the buffer hole R_d damage radius and spacing are:

- The calculated R_d is a starting point for design. The calculated result should be close to what will provide the best damage control result but should not be considered the absolute result.

- Trial blasts are suggested to optimize the controlled blast design.

- The MAE R_d damage model is a sound empirical approach for average rock conditions; R_d calculations from explosives used in the successful designs had in all cases, except in one, good correlation with actual R_d distances.

- Any R_d/r_h user results that are outside the range of 20 to 30 for buffer holes should be considered suspect. The range of R_d/r_h values used in the successful designs was 20.8 to 30.4.

- Buffer hole spacing is suggested within a range of 1.3 R_d to 1.5 R_d. This is a valid range because the successful designs vary from 1.1 R_d to 2.1 R_d. The lower end of the suggested range is recommended to provide closer spacing of the perimeter holes which are located at the cusps between buffer holes.

Guidance points relating to use of the proper perimeter hole charging and spacing are:

- The perimeter hole spacing is based on the buffer holes spacing.

- Charging of the perimeter based on Sanden [1974] will assure the user that a high enough hole pressure is used to split the perimeter in the event the buffer row did not damage the perimeter burden sufficiently.

- Perimeter hole spacing as described in the buffer row design method is suggested within a range of 1.3 R_d to 1.5 R_d which is the same as the buffer hole spacing. The successful designs' perimeter spacing varied from 1.0 R_d to1.4 R_d indicating that the suggested spacing should be closer to 1.3 R_d or even lower. In support for closer than

1.3 R_d spacing for the perimeter row is the point that the lowest buffer spacing in the successful designs was 1.1 R_d, which would result in equally close spacing for the perimeter holes if the buffer row concept was used. Further, the percentage of area covered by the buffer hole MAE R_d circles would be greater as the circle spacing decreases. A compromise in hole spacing to assure a successful controlled blast design that would accommodate both the buffer spacing and the perimeter spacing would be a narrow range around 1.3 R_d.

Conclusions

Overbreak is a concern in drift operations because of the associated loose rock, additional scaling requirements, and the increase in potential for fall-of-ground accidents. Excessive overbreak is a phenomenon that occurs because perimeter control is not generally applied. Today, available drilling and blasting technology has developed to the point that there is no reason why the rock mass cannot be "cut as with a knife", if so desired [Kvapil 2008]. A practical damage estimator R_d using the buffer row design method was presented as a solution to control the perimeter and reduce scaling requirements.

Three large block experiments confirmed the expected radial damage from fully coupled charges with measurements made both visually and with acoustic measurements. These tests confirm a close relationship between the practical damage radius R_d and the measured damage limits when applying the MAE approach.

The step-by-step algorithm for placement of buffer and perimeter holes was briefly described utilizing the R_d practical damage limit.

The practical damage estimator, R_d, was applied to actual successful perimeter control designs to affirm the use of the estimator for design. The estimator was shown to be valid in each example. It was found that the spacing of the buffer holes and the perimeter holes varies in the successful designs. A buffer design with buffer hole and perimeter hole spacings of 1.3 R_d is a good starting point and based on the successful designs.

The buffer row design concept provides a simple, and technically sound, method for assigning the damage radius for a particular explosive, hole diameter, and rock density combination.

Recommendations

Controlled blasting is recommended over aggressive blasting methods to reduce perimeter damage, scaling, and fall-of-ground accidents. The design, whether it is the buffer row concept described in this report or another design approach, must be engineered and implemented with the "buy-in" of the miner. Precision drilling is necessary to achieve as-drilled performance that is equal to as-designed performance. The jack leg drill cannot easily achieve this performance result; however, drill jumbos with precision control that can achieve as-designed results are recommended.

Deep mine stress and existing rock structure could affect the extent of blast damage. For example, the length of radial cracks could terminate at existing rock structure preventing further damage. High-stress conditions could alter the circular radial cracking pattern. Research into these areas is recommended.

Acknowledgments

The National Institute for Occupational Safety and Health (NIOSH) engineers who contributed to the controlled blasting research during the field studies and blast damage model development include Jami Dwyer, Douglas Tesarik, Joel Warneke, Edward McHugh, Chuck Kerkering, Yasser Akbarzedah, Rimas Pakalnis, Tom Brady, and Mark Kuchta. Publication outputs from the controlled blasting for safety project are listed in the Bibliography section following the References section. Other NIOSH technical staff who contributed to this research project includes Steve Ward, Ron Jackshaw, Mike Stepan, Paul Pierce, and Richard Rains. A special acknowledgment is given to the mines and their staff who provided information.

References

Ash, RL [1963a] The mechanics of rock breakage – part 1. Pit and Quarry 56(2):98–100.

Ash RL [1963b]. The mechanics of rock breakage – part 2: standards for blasting design. Pit and Quarry 56(3):118–122.

Ash RL [1963c]. The mechanics of rock breakage – part 3: the characteristics of explosives. Pit and Quarry 56(4):126–131.

Ash RL [1963d]. The mechanics of rock breakage – part 4: material properties, powder factor, blasting cost. Pit and Quarry 56(5):109–118.

Cudmore B [2001]. Perimeter blasting – an overview. Presented at the 15th Mine Operators Conference, The Canadian Institute of Mining – Mines Operations Centre (CIM-MOC), Saskatoon, SK, Canada, February 11–15, 2001, 10 pp.

Drukovanyi NF, Kravtsov VS, Chernyavskii YE, Shelenok VV, Reva NP, Zver'kov SN [1976]. Calculation of fracture zones created by exploding cylindrical charges in ledge rock. Soviet Mining Science 12(3):292–295.

Etkin MB, Azarkovich AE, Sapronov AA, and Vartanov VG [2001]. Protecting external rock bodies from blasting damage. Hydrotechnical Construction 35(9):499–506.

Fauske A [2003]. Practical experiences and possibilities using SSE string charging system. In: Holmberg R, ed. Explosives and Blasting Technique, Proceedings of the EFEE Second World Conference on Explosives and Blasting Technique, September 10–12, Prague, Czech Republic. A.A. Balkema Publishers, pp. 253–260.

Favreau RF [1969]. Generation of strain waves in rock by an explosion in a spherical cavity. J Geophys Res 74(4):267–4,280.

Holmberg R [1982]. Charge calculations for tunneling. Section 7.5: Blasting, Chapter 1. In: Hustrulid WA, ed. Underground mining methods handbook SME, pp. 1580–1589.

Holmberg R, Persson PA [1979]. Design of tunnel perimeter blasthole patterns to prevent rock damage. In: Jones MJ, ed. Proceedings of the Second International Symposium Tunnelling '79, London: Institution of Mining and Metallurgy, p. 280–283.

Hustrulid W [1999a]. Blasting principles for open pit mining, volume 1: general design concepts. Rotterdam, Netherlands: A.A.Balkema, 382 pp.

Hustrulid W [1999b]. Blasting principles for open pit mining, volume 2: theoretical foundations. Rotterdam, Netherlands: A.A.Balkema, 1,013 pp.

Hustrulid W [2007]. A practical, yet technically sound design procedure for pre-split blasts. In: Proceedings of the 33rd Annual Meeting, ISEE. Nashville, TN: Jan 28–31, 26 pp.

Hustrulid W [2008]. Perimeter control blasting in drifting—some new insights. Presented at the Northwest Mining Association's 114th Annual Meeting, Exposition and Short Courses – John Ascuaga's Nugget Casino Resort, Sparks, Nevada, "Mining for a Minerals Dependent World", December 1–5, 2008.

Hustrulid W [2010]. Some comments regarding development drifting practices with special emphasis on caving applications. In: Potvin, ed. Proceedings of Caving 2010, Perth, Australia: Australian Centre for Geomechanics, 44 pp.

Hustrulid W and Johnson J [2008]. A gas pressure-based drift round blast design methodology. In: Proceedings of the MassMin 2008, 5th International Conference & Exhibition on Mass Mining Technology. Luleå, Sweden, pp. 657–669.

Iannacchione AT and Prosser LJ [1997]. Roof and rib hazard assessment for underground stone mines. Society for Mining, Metallurgy, and Exploration, Inc. Preprint 97-11, Denver, Colorado, February 24–27, 1997, 5 pp.

Iverson SR, McHugh EL, Dwyer J, Warneke J, Caceres C [2007]. Ground control and safety implications of blast damage in underground mines, 26th International Conference on Ground Control in Mining, 9 pp.

Iverson SR, Hustrulid WA, Johnson JC, Tesarik D, Akbarzadeh Y [2009]. The extent of blast damage from a fully coupled explosive charge. In: Sanchidrián JA, ed. Proceedings of Rock Fragmentation by Blasting: 9th International Symposium On Rock Fragmentation by Blasting – Fragblast 9. Granada, Spain: CRC Press, pp. 459–468.

Johnson JC [2010]. The Hustrulid bar – a dynamic strength test and its application to the cautious blasting of rock [dissertation]. Salt Lake City, UT: University of Utah, Department of Mining Engineering.

Konya CJ [2006]. Rock blasting and overbreak control, 3rd ed. of U.S. Department of Transportation contract report DTFH 61-90-R-00058, Dec. 1991, 432 pp.

Kvapil R [2008]. Telephone conversation on January 2008 between R. Kvapil, retired, and William Hustrulid, Office of Mine Safety and Health Research, National Institute for Occupational Safety and Health, Centers for Disease Control, U.S. Department of Health and Human Services.

Markland P [2011]. (Per-Ivar.Marklund@boliden.com) [2011]. Private e-mail message to William Hustrulid (whustrulid@aol.com), February 2011.

Marshall GD, Sarin DK, Hampton VE [1983]. Work place ground support at Inco's Thompson Mine. In: Stability in Underground Mining, Chapter 41, First International Conference on Stability in Underground Mining, August 16–18, 1982, Vancouver, British Columbia, Canada: pp. 902–921.

McCarter M. K., [1996]. Effect of blast preconditioning on comminution for selected rock types. In: Proceedings of the Twenty-Second Conference of Explosives and Blasting Technique, Orlando, Florida, February 4–8, 1996. International Society of Explosives Engineers, Cleveland, Ohio, pp. 119–129.

McHugh E, Warneke J, Caceres C [2008a]. A case study examination of two blast rounds at a Nevada gold mine. The Journal of Explosives Engineers, November/December 2008, pp. 34–44.

McHugh E, Warneke J, Caceres C [2008b]. A case study examination of two blast rounds at a Nevada gold mine. In: Proceedings of the Thirty-Fourth Annual Conference on Explosives and Blasting Technique, International Society of Explosives Engineers, January 27–30, 2008. New Orleans, LA, 15 pp.

Neiman IB [1979]. Determination of the zone of crushing of rock in place by blasting. Soviet Mining Science, 15(5):pp. 480–499.

Norling L, Nord G [2006]. The blasting result in underground mine development and production using modern drill rigs. In: Proceedings of 8th International Symposia on Rock Fragmentation by Blasting – Fragblast 8. Santiago, Chile: May 7–11, 2006: pp. 365–368.

Persson PA, Holmberg R, Lee J [1994]. Rock blasting and explosives engineering. Boca Raton, FL: CRC Press, 540 pp.

Sanden BH [1974]. Presplit blasting [unpublished MSc. thesis]. Kingston, Ontario, Canada: Queen's University, Mining Engineering Department.

Sher EN [1997]. Taking into account the dynamics in description of fracture of brittle media by an explosion of a cord charge. J Appl Mech Tech Phys 38(3):484–492.

Sher EN, Aleksandrova NI [1997]. Dynamics of development of crushing zone in elasto plastic medium in camouflet explosion of string charge, J Min Sci 33(6):529–535.

Sher EN, Aleksandrova NI [2007]. Effect of borehole charge structure on the parameters of a failure zone in rocks under blasting. Journal of Mining Science 43(4):409–417.

Singh P, Narendrula R [2007]. The influence of rock mass quality in controlled blasting. In: Proceedings of the 26th International Conference on Ground Control in Mining, July 31–August 2. Morgantown, WV: 6 pp.

Sutherland M [1989]. Improving mine safety through perimeter blasting at Inco Limited's Thompson T-3 Mine, Ninth Underground Operators' Conference, Sudbury, Ontario, February 19–22, 6 pp.

Tesarik DR and Hustrulid WA [2009]. A hydrodynamics-based approach for predicting the blast damage zone in drifting as demonstrated using concrete block data. Blasting and Fragmentation Journal 3(2): 141–166.

Tesarik DR, Hustrulid WA, Nyberg U [2011]. Assessment and application of a single charge-blast test at the Kiruna mine, Sweden. Blasting and Fragmentation Journal 5(1):47–71.

Warneke J, Dwyer JG, Orr T [2007]. Use of a 3-D scanning laser to quantify drift geometry and overbreak due to blast damage in underground manned entries. In: Eberhardt E, Stead D, Morrison T, eds. Proceedings of the 1st Canada–US Rock Mechanics Symposium, May 27–31. Vancouver, Canada: pp. 93–100.

Project Bibliography

Dwyer J, Johnson J, Whyatt J, White B [2005]. Fragmentation method: a ground-control tool. Mining Engineering, March, 2005, pp. 37–42.

Hustrulid W [2007]. A practical, yet technically sound design procedure for pre-split blasts. In: Proceedings of the 33rd Annual Meeting, ISEE. Nashville, TN: Jan 28–31, 26 pp.

Hustrulid W, Johnson J [2008]. A gas pressure-based drift round blast design methodology. In: Proceedings of the Mass Min 2008, 5th International Conference & Exhibition on Mass Mining, Luleå, Sweden, pp. 657–669.

Hustrulid WA, Iverson SR [2009]. Evaluation of Kiruna mine drifting data using the NIOSH design approach. In: JA Sanchidrián, ed. Proceedings of Fragblast 9: Rock Fragmentation by Blasting, CRC Press, pp. 497–506.

Hustrulid W [2010]. Some comments regarding development drifting practices with special emphasis on caving applications. Caving 2010, Y. Potvin, ed. Australian Centre for Geomechanics, Perth, Australia, 44 pp.

Iverson SR, McHugh EL, Dwyer J, Warneke J, Caceres C [2007]. Ground control and safety implications of blast damage in underground mines. In: Proceedings of the 26th International Conference on Ground Control in Mining. Morgantown, WV, 9 pp.

Iverson SR, Kerkering C, Hustrulid W [2008]. Application of the NIOSH-modified Holmberg-Persson approach to perimeter blast design. In: Proceedings of the Thirty-Fourth Annual Conference on Explosives and Blasting Technique, International Society of Explosives Engineers, January 27–30, 2008, New Orleans, LA, 33 pp.

Iverson SR, Hustrulid WA, Johnson JC, Tesarik D, Akbarzadeh Y [2009]. The extent of blast damage from a fully coupled explosive charge. In: JA Sanchidrián, ed. Proceedings of Fragblast 9–Rock Fragmentation by Blasting. CRC Press, pp. 459–468.

Johnson J [2010]. The Hustrulid bar – a dynamic strength test and its application to the cautious blasting of rock [Ph.D. dissertation]. Salt Lake City, UT: University of Utah, 340 pp.

Johnson JC, Hustrulid WA [2009]. Measurement of the dynamic compressive strength of solids from the decay of strain in long bars. Society of Experimental Mechanics Symposium, Albuquerque, New Mexico, June 1–3, 2009.

Johnson JC, Hustrulid WA, Iverson SR [2009]. A method to calculate dynamic compressive stress damage in rock. 43rd U.S. Rock Mechanics Symposium. Asheville, North Carolina, June 28–July 1, 2009.

McHugh E, Warneke J, Caceres C [2008a]. A case study examination of two blast rounds at a Nevada gold mine. The Journal of Explosives Engineers, November/December 2008, pp. 34–44.

McHugh E, Warneke J, Caceres C [2008b]. A case study examination of two blast rounds at a Nevada gold mine. In: Proceedings of the Thirty-Fourth Annual Conference on Explosives and Blasting Technique, International Society of Explosives Engineers, January 27–30, 2008. New Orleans, LA, 15 pp.

Singer JA, Link CA, Iverson SR [2009]. High resolution seismic refraction tomography for determining depth of blast induced damage in a mine wall. Blasting and Fragmentation Journal 3(2):115–140.

Tesarik DR, Hustrulid WA [2009]. A hydrodynamics-based approach for predicting the blast damage zone in drifting as demonstrated using concrete block data. Blasting and Fragmentation Journal 3(2):141–166.

Tesarik DR, Hustrulid WA, Nyberg U [2011]. Assessment and application of a single charge-blast test at the Kiruna mine, Sweden. Blasting and Fragmentation Journal 5(1) May 2011, pp. 47–71.

Warneke J, Dwyer JG, Orr T [2007]. Use of a 3-D scanning laser to quantify drift geometry and overbreak due to blast damage in underground manned entries. In: Proceedings of the Vancouver Rock Mechanics Conference. 8 pp.

Whyatt J, Girard J, Johnson J [2003]. Feasibility of using controlled blasting techniques to improve ground control safety in underground mines. Proceedings, Soil and Rock America 2003, 12th Pan American Conference on Soil Mechanics and Geotechnical Engineering and 39th US Rock Mechanics Symposium, M.I.T., Cambridge, Massachusetts, June 22–26, 2003, Verlag Glückauf GmbH Essen, Vol. 2, 1717–1724.

Appendix A:

**Perimeter Hole Covolume Wall Pressure Calculation Method
Used for Successful Design Examples**

Perimeter Hole Covolume Wall Pressure Calculation Method Used for Successful Design Examples

The pressure on the borehole wall for decoupled charges is explained in Hustrulid and Johnson [2008]. Generally, the explosion pressures are much higher than the compressive strength of the rock being blasted. Although this is desired when fracturing the rock in the interior part of the drift round, it is not true for the perimeter holes when perimeter control blasting is to be used.

The first design requirement for these holes is to keep the borehole wall pressure less than or equal to the unconfined compressive strength. This is normally accomplished by using decoupled charges. The explosion pressure applies at the outer boundary of the charge. To reach the borehole wall, the explosive gases must expand.

For ideal gases (gases at atmospheric pressure and room temperature), the standard expression relating pressure, volume, and temperature is

$$Pv = nRT \qquad (19)$$

where P = pressure,

v = specific volume,

n = number of moles of gas present,

T = temperature, and

R = the Universal Gas Constant.

Assuming isothermal expansion, one writes

$$P_w v_h = P_e v_e \qquad (20)$$

where P_e = explosion pressure,

v_e = specific volume of the explosive,

P_w = wall pressure, and

v_h = specific volume of explosive gases filling the hole.

Assume that

$$\rho_e = 0.82 \text{ g/cm}^3$$

The specific volume of the explosive would be

$$v_e = 1/\rho_e = 1/0.82 = 1.22 \text{ cm}^3/\text{g} \tag{21}$$

For the case when d_h = hole diameter = 54 mm and

d_e = explosive diameter = 30 mm,

the specific volume of the gases filling the hole is given by

$$v_h = \left(\frac{d_h}{d_e}\right)^2 v_e = \left(\frac{54}{30}\right)^2 1.22 = 3.95 \text{ L/kg} \tag{22}$$

Applying Equation 20 and assuming an explosion pressure of 1560 MPa, the wall pressure would be

$$P_w = P_e\left(\frac{v_e}{v_h}\right) = 1,560\left(\frac{1.22}{3.95}\right) = 482 \text{ MPa} \tag{23}$$

However, one cannot apply this approach for the very high-pressure, high-temperature explosive gases involved here. The relationship relating pressure, volume, and temperature is:

$$P(v - \alpha) = nRT \tag{24}$$

where P = pressure (atm),

v = specific volume (L/kg),

α = covolume (L/kg),

n = moles/kg,

R = universal gas constant = 0.08207 L-atm/(K-mol), and

T = temperature (K).

The expression

$$\alpha_h = 1.1e^{-0.473/v} \tag{25}$$

will be used to relate the covolume and the specific volume. Assuming as before that the expansion of the gases in the borehole occurs isothermally, one can write

$$P_w(v_h - \alpha_h) = P_e(v_e - \alpha_e) \tag{26}$$

where

$$\alpha_h = 1.1e^{-0.473/v_h} \tag{27}$$

$$\alpha_e = 1.1e^{-0.473/v_e} \tag{28}$$

Substituting the appropriate values, one finds that

$$\alpha_h = 1.1e^{-0.473/v_h} = 1.1e^{-0.473/3.95} = 0.976$$

$$\alpha_e = 1.1e^{-0.473/v_e} = 1.1e^{-0.473/1.22} = 0.718$$

The wall pressure with the covolume correction becomes

$$P_w = P_e \left(\frac{(v_e - \alpha_e)}{(v_h - \alpha_h)} \right) = 1,560 \left(\frac{1.22 - 0.502}{3.95 - 2.974} \right) = 263 \text{ MPa}$$

As can be seen, the covolume correction has a major effect. If the compressive strength is, for example,

$$\sigma_c = 200 \text{ MPa}$$

one would expect to see crushing around the hole.

Table 20. Covolume spreadsheet calculation for Australian design

Covolume calculation	Value	Units	Notes	Formula
dh	0.048	m	Blasthole diameter	None
de	0.034	m	Explosive diameter	None
Evod	4.3	km/sec	Velocity of detonation for the explosive	None
Edensity	850	kg/m^3	Density of the explosive	None
v_e	1.176471	--	Specific volume of explosive	1/(Edensity/1,000)
Ve	0.440629	--	Volume term	v_e-1.1*EXP(−0.473/v_e)
vh_	2.3448	--	Explosive gas specific volume	v_e*(dh/de)^2
Vh	1.445746	--	Volume term	vh_-1.1*EXP(−0.473/vh_)
Pewall	598	MPa	Wall pressure from decoupled charge	1/8*Edensity*Evod^2*(Ve/Vh)
Coupled pressure	1,965	MPa	Wall pressure if fully coupled	1/8*Edensity*Evod^2

Table 21. Covolume spreadsheet calculation for bottom charge design

Covolume calculation	Value	Units	Notes	Formula
dh	0.048	m	Blasthole diameter	None
de	0.014	m	Explosive diameter	None
Evod	3.9	km/sec	Velocity of detonation for the explosive	None
Edensity	950	kg/m^3	Density of the explosive	None
v_e	1.052632	--	Specific volume of explosive	1/(Edensity/1,000)
Ve	0.350785	--	Volume term	v_e-1.1*EXP(−0.473/v_e)
vh_	12.37379	--	Explosive gas specific volume	v_e*(dh/de)^2
Vh	11.31505	--	Volume term	vh_-1.1*EXP(−0.473/vh_)
Pewall	56	MPa	Wall pressure from decoupled charge	1/8*Edensity*Evod^2*(Ve/Vh)
Coupled pressure	1,806	MPa	Wall pressure if fully coupled	1/8*Edensity*Evod^2

Table 22. Covolume spreadsheet calculation for Swedish decoupled design

Covolume calculation	Value	Units	Notes	Formula
dh	0.048	m	Blasthole diameter	None
de	0.017	m	Explosive diameter	None
Evod	2.4	km/sec	Velocity of detonation for the explosive	None
Edensity	1,000	kg/m^3	Density of the explosive	None
v_e	1	--	Specific volume of explosive	1/(Edensity/1,000)
Ve	0.314557	--	Volume term	v_e-1.1*EXP(−0.473/v_e)
vh_	7.972318	--	Explosive gas specific volume	v_e*(dh/de)^2
Vh	6.935683	--	Volume term	vh_-1.1*EXP(−0.473/vh_)
Pewall	33	MPa	Wall pressure from decoupled charge	1/8*Edensity*Evod^2*(Ve/Vh)
Coupled pressure	720	MPa	Wall pressure if fully coupled	1/8*Edensity*Evod^2

Table 23. Covolume spreadsheet calculation for Canadian design

Covolume calculation	Value	Units	Notes	Formula
dh	0.045	m	Blasthole diameter	None
de	0.022	m	Explosive diameter	None
Evod	7	km/sec	Velocity of detonation for the explosive	None
Edensity	1,300	kg/m^3	Density of the explosive	None
v_e	0.769231	--	Specific volume of explosive	1/(Edensity/1,000)
Ve	0.174466	--	Volume term	v_e-1.1*EXP(−0.473/v_e)
vh_	3.218373	--	Explosive gas specific volume	v_e*(dh/de)^2
Vh	2.268719	--	Volume term	vh_-1.1*EXP(−0.473/vh_)
Pewall	612	MPa	Wall pressure from decoupled charge	1/8*Edensity*Evod^2*(Ve/Vh)
Coupled pressure	7,963	MPa	Wall pressure if fully coupled	1/8*Edensity*Evod^2

Table 24. Covolume spreadsheet calculation for Spanish design

Covolume calculation	Value	Units	Notes	Formula
dh	0.045	m	Blasthole diameter	None
de	0.0095	m	Explosive diameter	None
Evod	7	km/sec	Velocity of detonation for the explosive	None
Edensity	1,400	kg/m^3	Density of the explosive	None
v_e	0.714286	--	Specific volume of explosive	1/(Edensity/1,000)
Ve	0.146999	--	Volume term	v_e-1.1*EXP(−0.473/v_e)
vh_	16.02691	--	Explosive gas specific volume	v_e*(dh/de)^2
Vh	14.9589	--	Volume term	vh_-1.1*EXP(−0.473/vh_)
Pewall	84	MPa	Wall pressure from decoupled charge	1/8*Edensity*Evod^2*(Ve/Vh)
Coupled pressure	8,575	MPa	Wall pressure if fully coupled	1/8*Edensity*Evod^2